W9-ATY-498

THE HEALING LABYRINTH

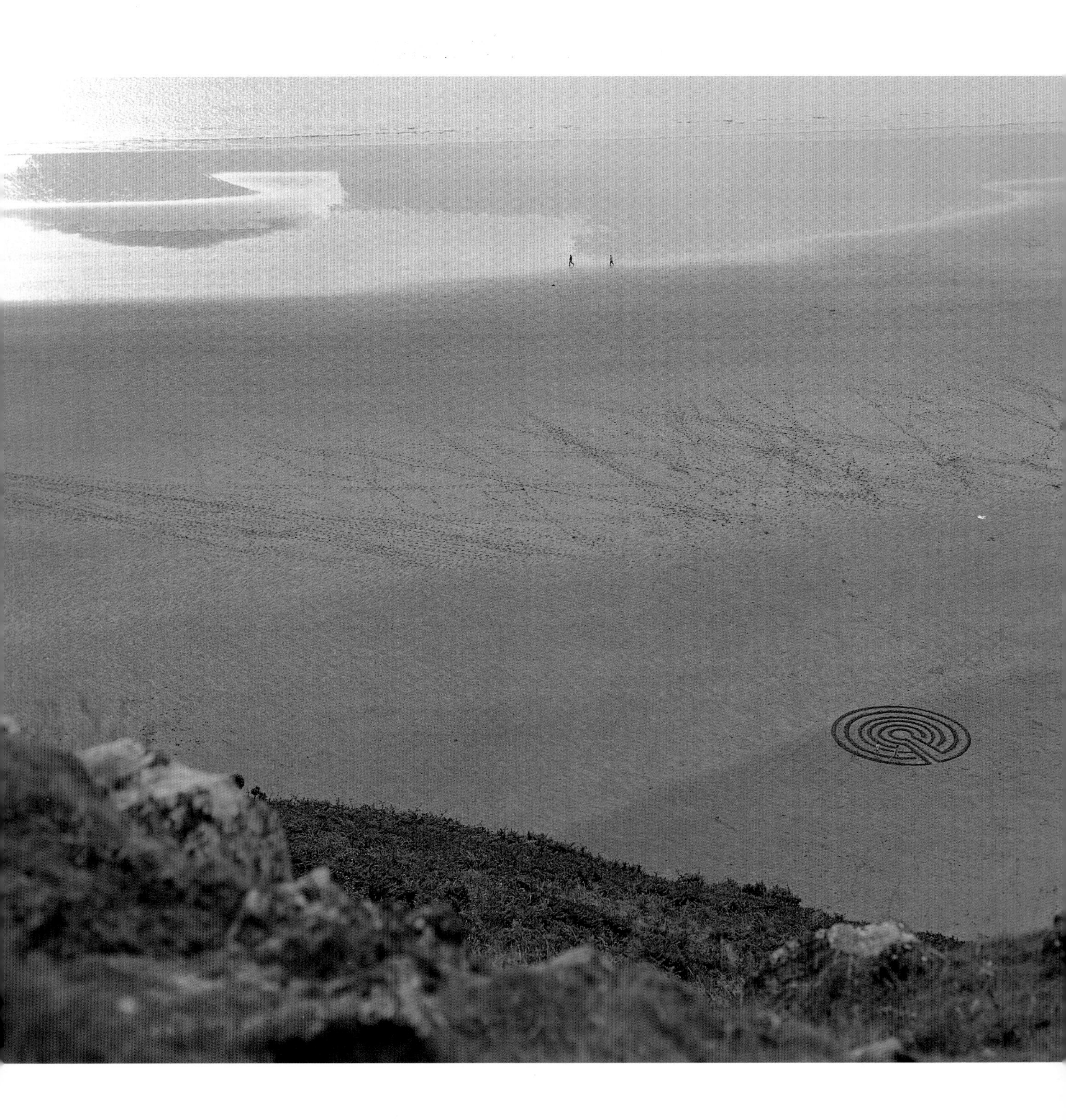

The Healing Labyrinth

Helen Raphael Sands

Foreword by Robert Ferré

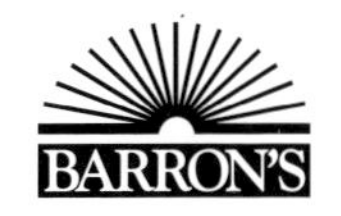

United States edition © 2001 by Barron's Educational Series, Inc.
First edition for the United States and Canada published 2001 by
Barron's Educational Series, Inc.

All inquiries should be addressed to:
Barron's Educational Series, Inc.
250 Wireless Boulevard
Hauppauge, New York 11788
http://www.barronseduc.com

Library of Congress Catalog Card No.00-105778
International Standard Book No. 0-7641-5325-0

Printed in Italy

9 8 7 6 5 4 3 2 1

Opposite: Medieval Mizmaze on top of St. Catherine's Hill near Winchester, England.
Page 2: Classical labyrinth drawn into sand at Rhossilli Bay in Wales.

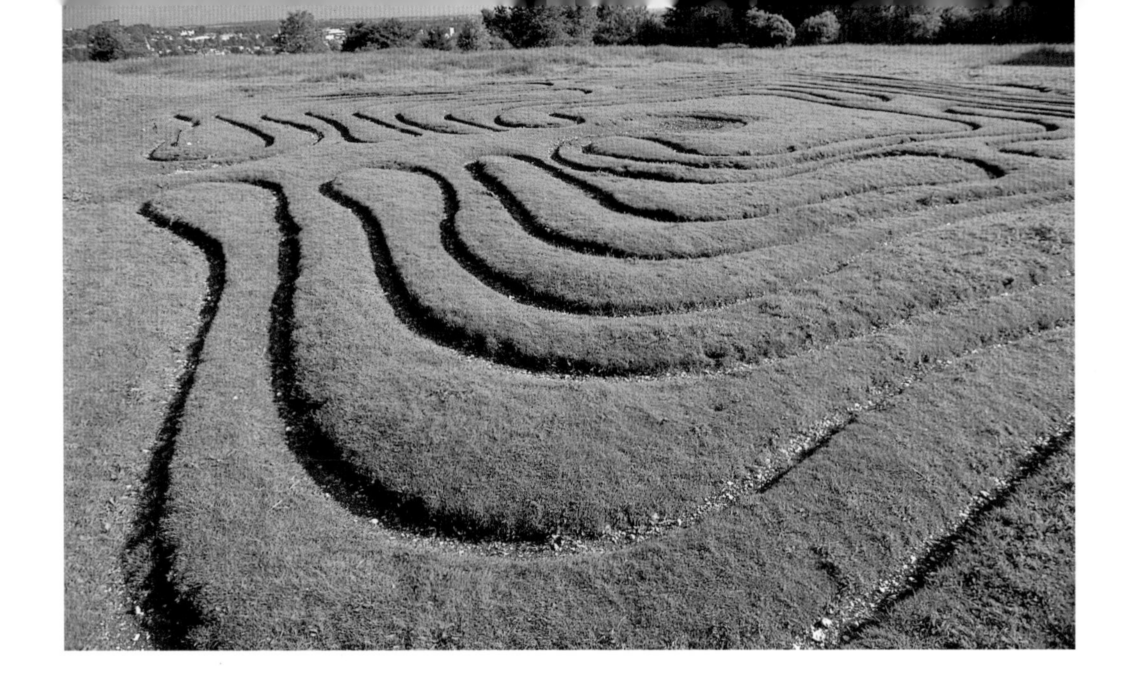

contents

Robert Ferré is a full-time labyrinth maker and tour director of One Heart Tours, which specializes in pilgrimage to sacred sites in France, notably Chartres. He is author of several labyrinth manuals and also supplies the canvas labyrinths sold by Veriditas at Grace Cathedral, San Francisco. He lives with his wife near St. Louis, Missouri.

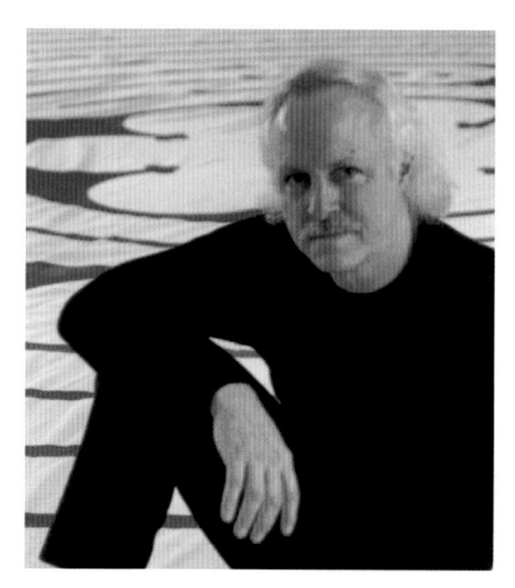

Foreword

Walking a labyrinth is an intensely personal endeavor. There is nothing that is supposed to happen. Indeed, no one can predict what experience the labyrinth will generate. The labyrinth is like a great magnifier, homing in on aspects of our lives that are often unconscious and making them apparent. If you want to understand your experience on the labyrinth, pay attention to the ways in which it reflects your own values, beliefs, and issues. Look within.

It is the personal nature of labyrinths that comes through so clearly in Helen Raphael Sands' beautiful book. She tells us her story and what the labyrinth has meant on her journey. Her life serves more as a metaphor than a biography, showing us the possibilities that are available to each of us—not to copy her, but to find our own way. To make it easier, she gives us helpful instruction, so that we have a context for understanding and framing our own experiences.

In all spiritual traditions there is some mechanism designed to get us beyond the surface, beyond appearance, opinion and conditioning, beyond ego, illusion and intellect, beyond imitation and personality. Real freedom lies in going deeper and arriving not at some foreign or unfamiliar place, but at ourselves, our wise, innocent, and loving selves. There we find healing and forgiveness and unlimited potential. This is our true destination—and the labyrinth can take us there.

Did I just say that we can encounter our authentic selves simply by walking a labyrinth? Oh, yes! All of us who work with labyrinths are continuously surprised by the variety, depth, and relevance of the experiences reported to us. In this way Helen Raphael Sands' story is not unique, for anyone who decides to follow its path will embark on their own journey. Can we conduct our pilgrimage alone? Sure! But it's a lot easier and more fun with a guide and as such Helen is poetic, sensitive, and honest. She leads without pulling and encourages without pushing. Asking us to do nothing that she hasn't done herself, she points us in the right direction, dancing all the way home.

Robert Ferré

Robert Ferré
August 2000

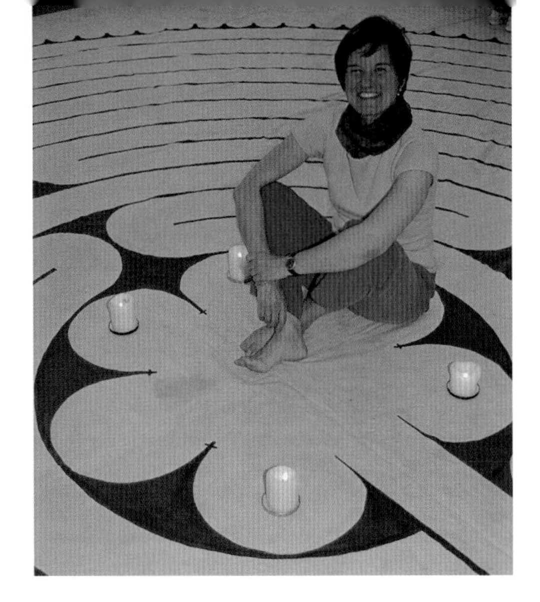

I dedicate this book to my father, Frederick John Frodsham, and my mother, Maria Matilda Schenk, with whom the dancing adventure on the labyrinth began.

How to use this book

The introduction offers the story of my encounter with labyrinths, in particular the one found on the stone floor in Chartres Cathedral in France. It is both an account of how I became involved with labyrinths and an example of how they can touch and change lives. Chapter One looks at labyrinths from a historical perspective and investigates why this ancient symbol holds such universal appeal. What follows this is an exploration of the journey on the labyrinth. For the purpose of the book I have organized it into three stages that have emerged from my own experience of running workshops. "Preparing the Ground" shows you how to activate your energy and the energy latent in the labyrinth before you follow the path to the center. It suggests methods using music, movement, and ritual to locate the labyrinth in the three dimensions of space, time, and among people. "Journey to the Heart" offers you guidance on how to make your journey on the labyrinth and shares other pilgrims' experiences. "Grounding in the Present" looks at ways of bringing your experience to a close, while honoring what you may have found on the labyrinth. Finally, Chapter Five shows you how to create your own labyrinth. I would recommend that you start with simple designs using a pen and paper to trace with your finger. From there, you can progress to making a large-scale labyrinth to walk, run, or dance. There are also more ambitious and time-consuming ideas, including how to make a full-size Chartres labyrinth. Whatever design or size of labyrinth you choose to make, I wish you joy in the making and in the journeying.

Helen Raphael Sands

Helen Raphael Sands
August 2000

my path with the Labyrinth

Beginnings

Every day is a journey,
and the journey itself
is home.
Matsuo Bashō

My first memory of working with labyrinths belongs to the sea and her constant presense, her rhythmical movement, her ebbing, and flowing. In the late seventies I found myself on a deserted beach with a group of adults with learning difficulties, their friends, and their parents. With sticks and lengths of rope we endeavored to trace a labyrinth pattern on the damp, firm sand for fun. I remember buying a booklet on the labyrinth in Chartres Cathedral, France, at a mind, body, spirit festival in London, England. There was something about the complex design on the front cover that gripped my imagination. On the beach that day I tried to make sense of its twists and turns while shouting instructions to the desultory band of followers. We had just completed it and begun to make our journey through it, when the relentless tide came in, washing part of it, then half of it, then all of it away. With our efforts erased, we could but laugh, have a cup of tea, and call it a day. Yet the memory was there and the work had begun.

A few years later I made another labyrinth, this time chalking it out on the rough surface of an elementary school playground. The children dashed in and out with enthusiasm, and the white coiling pathways lasted a few days until their feet rubbed all trace of them away. Similarly, the image of the labyrinth faded from my mind through the eighties, absorbed as I was in my growing family and my work at a L'Arche community for adults with learning disabilities. In some ways I was asleep and protected in a way of life I thought would continue indefinitely. However, there was deep revolt and distress stirring inside me: some things just didn't fit anymore.

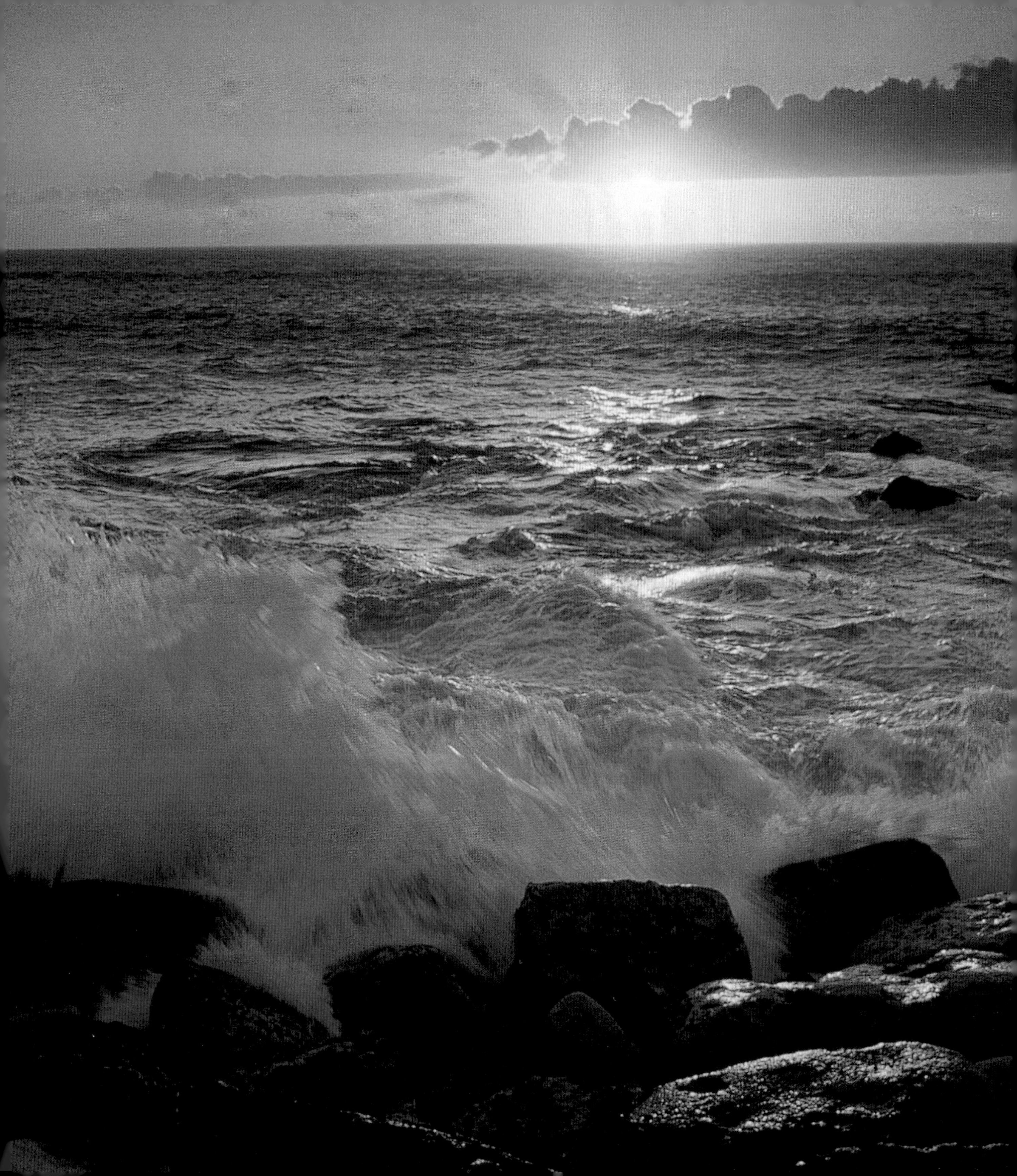

The catalyst was giving birth to my two daughters. This changed my whole being. Although filled with joy and energy, I also felt the demands of motherhood. At church—I was brought up a Christian in the Catholic tradition—the crying child, both inside me and in the form of my baby, was relegated to a crying chapel at the back of the church, so the other worshippers would not be disturbed. I felt my experience as a woman and as a mother was excluded by the patriarchal Church. I could not relate to Mary, Mother of Christ, who seemed too serene, remote, and queenly. I found that other women I met felt the same. I began to search for new words to voice my rage and joy, for new forms to express my being.

Two groups helped me to break free: I joined the Christian Parity Group in the early days of the Movement for the Ordination of Women and absorbed the stories women told as we sat in a circle; I also stumbled on Sacred Circle Dance during a chance visit to the Findhorn Community in Scotland. The rhythmic music and traditional dances touched my heart and stirred my subconscious. The steps seemed familiar, and Greek music in particular took me back to the ancient roots of ritual movement.

I drew hope and comfort from the sea that washed away the marks of yesterday to make way for the new. Rebuilt after a terrible fire in 1194, Chartres Cathedral in France (far right), viewed here from the northeast, was the inspiration for my journey with the labyrinth.

A life dismantled; a life regained

From the unreal lead me to the real.
From darkness lead me to light.
From death lead me to immortality.
The Upanishads

And then the crash came: my marriage collapsed at the end of the eighties and my involvement with the L'Arche community ended. Everything I trusted was swept away, except for life with my two children and the love of good friends. I flailed about in pain for a number of years until I felt a memory pulling and a great desire surfacing to make the journey to see the labyrinth in Chartres Cathedral. Without knowing it, I had my hand on a strong rope and it was pulling me in to dry land and new life.

The summer of 1995 was also the summer before my divorce. I was on holiday with my younger daughter and friends, passing the days in a house overlooking the sea in Normandy, France. Every night I could hear the waves flowing in over the beach, and every morning I could see the expanse of sand swept clean and pure before it was marked by new footprints. I felt the promise of being cleansed and having the detritus of recent years washed away. I took three shells from the shore, and set out for Chartres across the hot and dusty plains in a little car packed tight with two adults, their tempers short, and two children, whining in the back. We arrived and, as I crossed the threshold of the cathedral, walking out of the sun and into the arching darkness of that great space, my stomach kicked: I was home. Home in the Great Mother, *Notre Dame*. I cried and cried, and let the jeweled light of the stained glass fall on me. In the days that followed, I began to explore the cathedral dedicated to Our Lady. I found there were stories in the stained-glass windows, statues with compassionate faces, and old, worn stones showing the passage of ancestors. I left my shells at the foot of Our Lady of the Pillar and told her of the pain of the last years.

I found the labyrinth by the west door, covered by crowded ranks of chairs and hidden from view. I sat on the altar steps, my feet itching to dance and trace the coils of the labyrinth. My frustration led to an idea: perhaps I could make the shape of the labyrinth on something portable, thereby releasing it from its prison; perhaps other people would like to dance with it too. As we left Chartres in the twilight and raced back over the plains to the sea, great storm clouds were gathering. Cords of lightning flashed between the darkening sky and sea, and thunder crashed above us. I felt alive and happy. My first pilgrimage to Chartres had been made and an idea for another kind of pilgrimage—a journey with the labyrinth rolled up like a carpet—was germinating deep inside me.

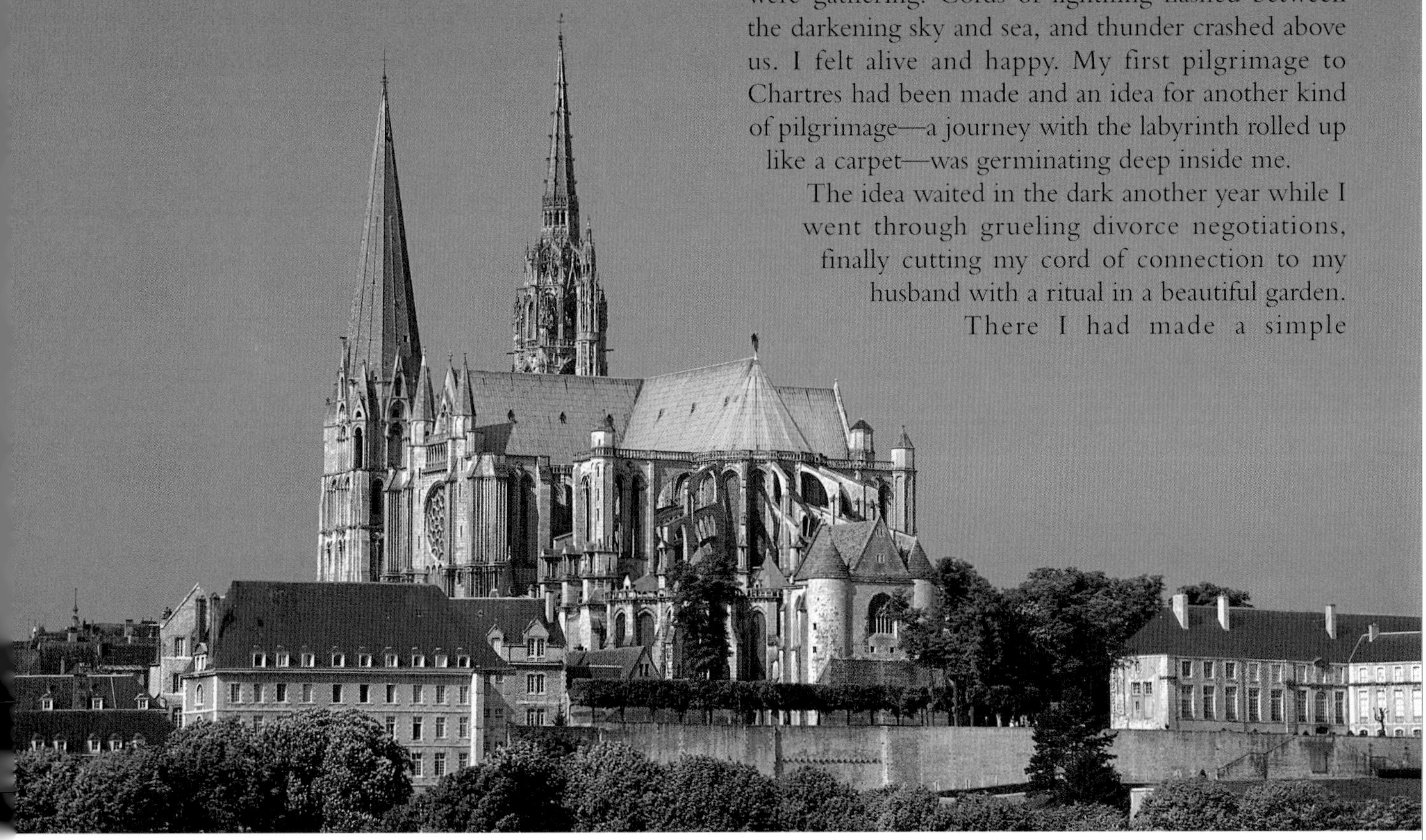

The idea waited in the dark another year while I went through grueling divorce negotiations, finally cutting my cord of connection to my husband with a ritual in a beautiful garden. There I had made a simple labyrinth with string. One behind the other we walked to the center, where we said good-bye with a song before treading our separate journeys out again.

In the summer of 1996 I went on another journey, driving from the south of England to the northeast of Scotland, to join a celebration of Sacred Circle Dance at the Findhorn community. I met many incredible people there, in particular a French woman named Geneviève who taught Circle Dance in Paris and was full of charm and laughter. She encouraged me to plan a millennium project, which would bring together dance and the labyrinth at numerous sacred and secular sites throughout Great Britain and Ireland. This would culminate in a joint Anglo-French pilgrimage to Chartres. At the close of the year I drew another sand labyrinth near Land's End in Cornwall. Treading it as darkness fell, I found Ariadne's thread (see p. 32) pulling and guiding me out of the ruins of my old life and into the unknown. I decided to make a long thread to accompany the labyrinth, which I would string with the names of all the places visited. Chartres would be the final destination.

Embarking on the journey

The first year of the pilgrimage with the portable labyrinth was a year of discovery. After much mathematical calculation and decision, I had a strong, 23-foot-wide, square canvas sewn together at a theatrical and artists' supplier in London. I had to reduce the labyrinth to just over half the size of the original in Chartres, as I wanted it to fit into average-sized indoor venues while preserving pathways of a reasonable width. Soon a friend and I were on our knees, penciling the concentric pathways on to the canvas. The outline complete, a small group of us painted the lines. I remember our aching knees and backs, the rasp of paintbrushes and pencils on the rough canvas and, finally, the swish of the broom as we swept it clean.

A few weeks later we laid out the pristine square canvas for the first time. Moving around each of the four sides, we dedicated it to the four elements (Earth, Air, Fire, and Water) from the Celtic tradition, the four directions (north, south, east, and west) from the Native American tradition and four archangels (Uriel, Gabriel, Raphael, and Michael) from the Christian tradition. Each of these added strength to the work of the canvas and breadth to its appeal. We danced a Circle Dance for each of the elements and, sitting

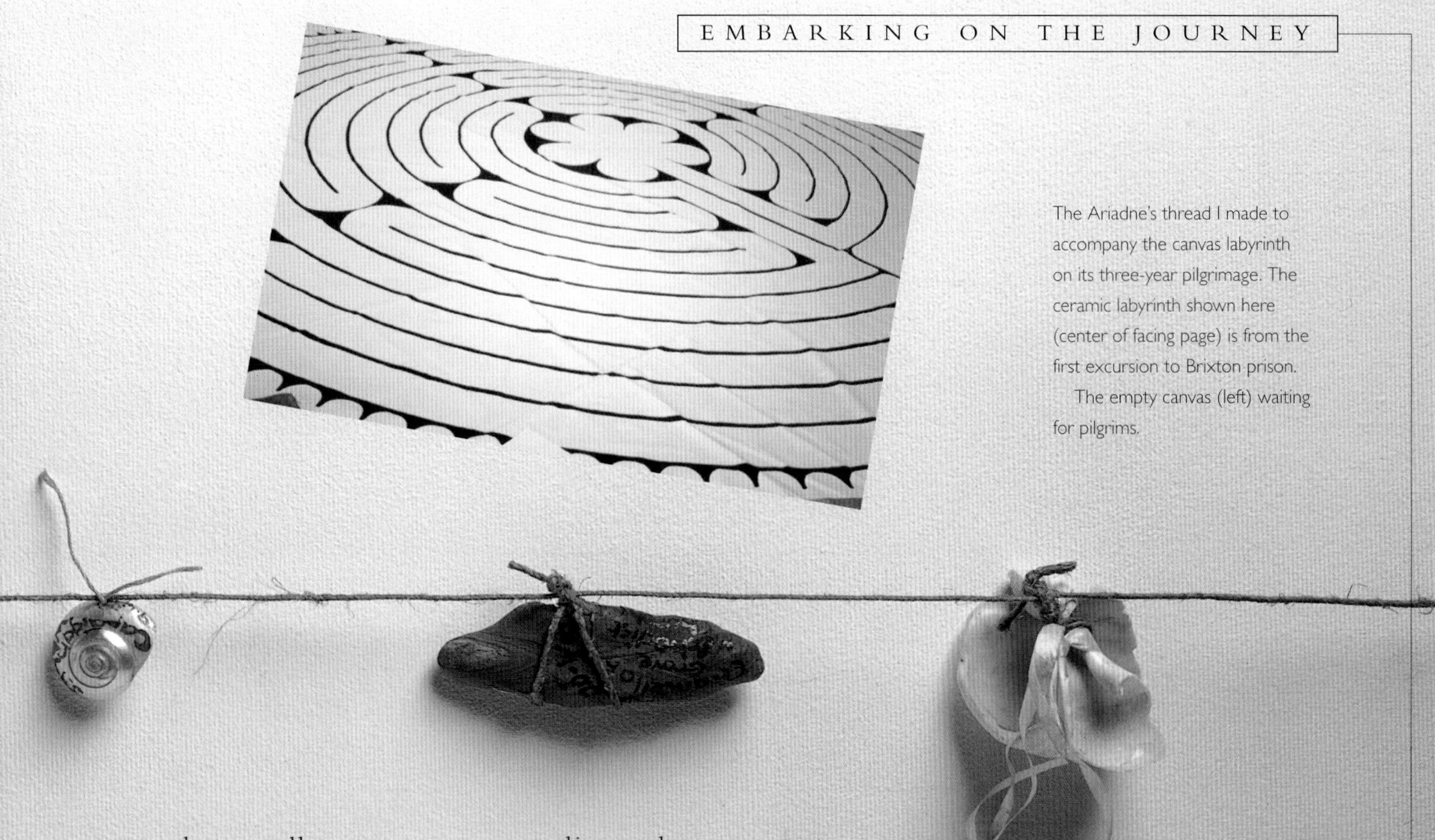

The Ariadne's thread I made to accompany the canvas labyrinth on its three-year pilgrimage. The ceramic labyrinth shown here (center of facing page) is from the first excursion to Brixton prison.

The empty canvas (left) waiting for pilgrims.

around a candle on one corner, listened to stories from the mists of time. I was beginning to learn what made the canvas come alive. As the work evolved a dialogue between opposites—the masculine and feminine, Heaven and Earth, the prehistoric and the Christian—seemed to emerge.

The labyrinth was first invited to Brixton prison in south London during Holy Week. The canvas looked completely at home as it lay in the chapel. I was tense, not knowing what to expect. The first man careened across the pathways wildly, so I took his hand to help him. Later, there were so many men clustered on one side of the canvas I thought the labyrinth was a ship that would tip and sink. But the ship proved a strong vessel, and the men found their way to the center and back again. The pilgrimage had begun.

Soon after I took the canvas to Ballydehob in Ireland for a women's drumming weekend. There we drummed and danced with the labyrinth to celebrate May Day. I was glad that with these first two venues the labyrinth was weaving together opposites: the imprisoned masculine at Brixton and the wild feminine in Ireland.

I soon found that by walking and dancing the labyrinth in certain locations, springs of blocked-up and forgotten energy could be released, both in and under the earth. On one occasion I took part in a ceremony to open an old bricked-up well. As the bricks fell away, water began to flow again. The next day we laid the labyrinth in a nearby field, where condensation left its imprint on the grass. The newly flowing spring water and the rippling lines of the labyrinth imprint seemed one and the same: they were both signs of released energy.

I began to learn more about strong currents of earth energy running through the landscape, often connecting places of special power and beauty. One such current spans England from the far west in Cornwall to the east coast in Norfolk. It is said to be made up of two snaking lines of energy, the Michael and Mary currents, with sacred sites at their intersection points (facing page, far right). One of these is at Glastonbury. I felt a strong urge to bring the labyrinth there and, in August of 1997, I laid it near the altar of the abbey ruins (below), where the two lines cross. Many people came to tread it, testing my ability to guide large groups. It was at once a magical and chaotic evening.

I learned of another line of earth energy, the Grail Line, originating in the south of France and running up through Chartres Cathedral (facing page, near right). After crossing the English Channel the line can be traced through west London, continuing up the spine of England and ending in Scotland. The island of Iona on the west coast of Scotland lies near it, home of St. Columba, who came there from Ireland in A.D. 563. I took the labyrinth there with a few pilgrims and laid it beside the small abbey. Huge skies, sunlight, a glimmering sea, and white sands heightened the experience. It was a place to shed the cares of the city and live simply; it was a paradise. As we followed the meandering path of the labyrinth we wove a dialectic between Celtic Christianity and its love of Nature and small homely rituals, and the grand flourish and style of medieval Christianity as expressed in the cathedral of Chartres.

With our footsteps we trod stories of simple Celtic saints into the labyrinth, such as St. Columba and St. Brigid of Ireland. According to legend, Brigid came to Iona and welcomed Mary into her house for the birth of Christ. In her pre-Christian form she is Triple Goddess—Maiden, Mother, and Crone—of poetry, smithcraft, and healing. Her part in the legend is a metaphor for the pre-Christian era, helping to give birth to the Christian era. Her face is an earlier form of the feminine archetype manifest in Mary.

Fear of the center

As I walked home one evening at the end of 1997 I was mugged. The violence was a great shock and stopped me in my tracks: it was a signal that the healing process that had begun with the labyrinth had to deepen to another level of my being. It was time to look inside at patterns of abuse I had carried since childhood. Life suddenly lost its luster and the joy recaptured over recent months disappeared. I went to Wales, turning to the sea and strength of the earth for healing. I felt I was being led to the heart of the labyrinth and to my heart within, where I had to meet my worst fears: inactivity; silence; the void. What lay in the space at the center of the labyrinth? Was it empty? Did it hold anything at all?

Just as Theseus in Ancient Greek mythology (see p. 32) had to thread through the labyrinth at Knossos to meet and kill the Minotaur in the center, so too did I have to enter this silence alone. Theseus held an

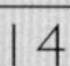

unraveled cord in his hand, which had been given to him by Ariadne, King Minos' daughter, so he could find his way back to the entrance. My cord was the love of friends and regular conversation with a counselor, all of whom helped me to walk back step by step into the world. For a few months the labyrinth lay dormant. I had put myself under pressure to organize events with it, but I slowly began to realize that my work with the labyrinth would unfold of its own accord, almost without me. All I had to do was follow the single, or unicursal, path to the center and out again. The journey would reveal lost memories and reconnect the layers from the past in a new wholeness.

I revisited Glastonbury and placed the labyrinth at three powerful sites: the first in view of the thorn tree on Wearyall Hill, where Joseph of Arimathea, follower of Jesus, is said to have planted his staff; the second by the spring in the Chalice Well gardens; the third, inside the abbey ruins, on the Mary energy line by the Lady Chapel, dedicated to the Virgin Mary. It was a joyful experience dancing there in the sunlight in the middle of the labyrinth and an important healing moment. As I danced to the music, my weaving, curling arms expressed my whole womanhood and the joy of my sexuality. I felt alive, and my feeling of exclusion from the Church was beginning to heal.

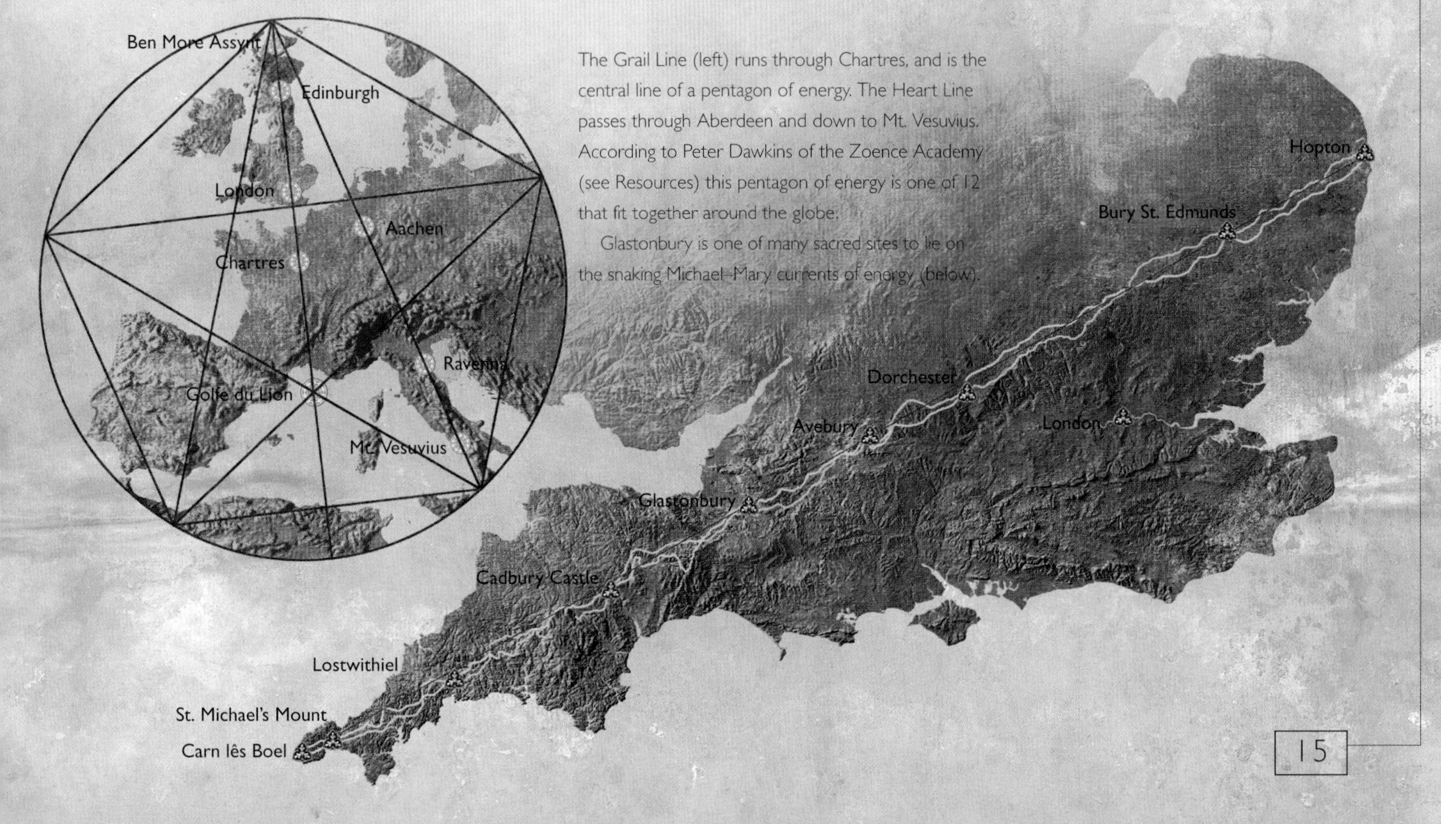

The Grail Line (left) runs through Chartres, and is the central line of a pentagon of energy. The Heart Line passes through Aberdeen and down to Mt. Vesuvius. According to Peter Dawkins of the Zoence Academy (see Resources) this pentagon of energy is one of 12 that fit together around the globe.

Glastonbury is one of many sacred sites to lie on the snaking Michael–Mary currents of energy (below).

Journeying out of the void

My confidence with the labyrinth grew. I discovered how the canvas could be brought to life with different kinds of music, as if the circuits of a labyrinth were like sound waves rippling out from the center. I choreographed new dances to echo the energy and mythology of each place we visited. At Avebury in Wiltshire, England, I used Hungarian folk music with a haunting woman's voice to celebrate the beauty and strength of the prehistoric stone circle.

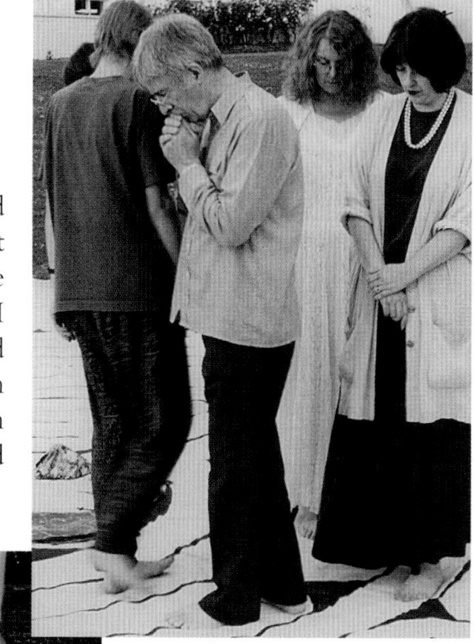

Celebrating my 50th birthday with a Mass on the labyrinth.

That year I continued to travel with the labyrinth. I visited Paris, returning the labyrinth to its country of origin, as well as locations in Wales and the north, west, and east of England. In London I laid the labyrinth beside the River Thames and worked with a theater company of young, homeless people. They walked the labyrinth as a *rite-de-passage*, marking the end of one production and the beginning of another.

On a personal level I was overcoming many past experiences, like a snake shedding its skin. Shadowy ghosts troubling me about my relationships with the masculine, specifically with my father, were laid to rest. I celebrated my 50th birthday with a Mass on the labyrinth. We arranged the gifts of bread and wine in the center of the labyrinth, and our offertory meditation was treading the labyrinth, finding the gifts, and bringing them out to be consecrated. That summer I visited Greece and I saw a production in the ancient, open-air amphitheater of Epidaurus. Nearby, in the healing sanctuary of Asclepius, God of Healing, I was drawn to the underground remains of a building called the *Tholos*, whose concentric walls and offset doorways reminded me of a labyrinth. Its use is unknown, though it may have been connected with sacred rites in the neighboring *Abato* building. Here the sick came and incubated a healing dream. At

Epidaurus I realized that walking coiling, labyrinthine pathways in the dark had been part of a healing process since ancient times, reflecting my own experience of interior darkness the previous year and the healing journey of rest and silence that I received at the heart of the labyrinth.

As autumn came, I felt I wanted to clear my life of past burdens and hurt, just as the wind clears the trees of leaves: I emptied cupboards and drawers; I attended the funerals of my former in-laws; my elder daughter left home for a journey around the world; and my former husband remarried. I felt stripped bare and found myself facing the empty space at the center of the labyrinth once more—what lay there? Deep down I knew that the end of the 20th century and the end of my old life would bring renewed joy and vision.

Passage to new life

I crossed the threshold of the 21st century outdoors in the Chalice Well gardens at Glastonbury. The symbol of the garden is called a *vesica piscis* and decorates the wooden cover of the well. It is a basic shape of sacred geometry and means "fish's bladder." It is formed with two intersecting circles and symbolizes the marriage of opposites, such as Heaven and Earth, the masculine and feminine, light and dark, not unlike the Chinese yin and yang symbol. That night in the calm of the garden, I felt Chalice Well was the intersection point of a huge imaginary *vesica piscis* drawn over the two other sites of celebration: to the northwest the abbey ruins housed a nocturnal ecumenical service with song and fireworks; to the east 700 flares were planted up the Tor hill to light the snaking procession of a

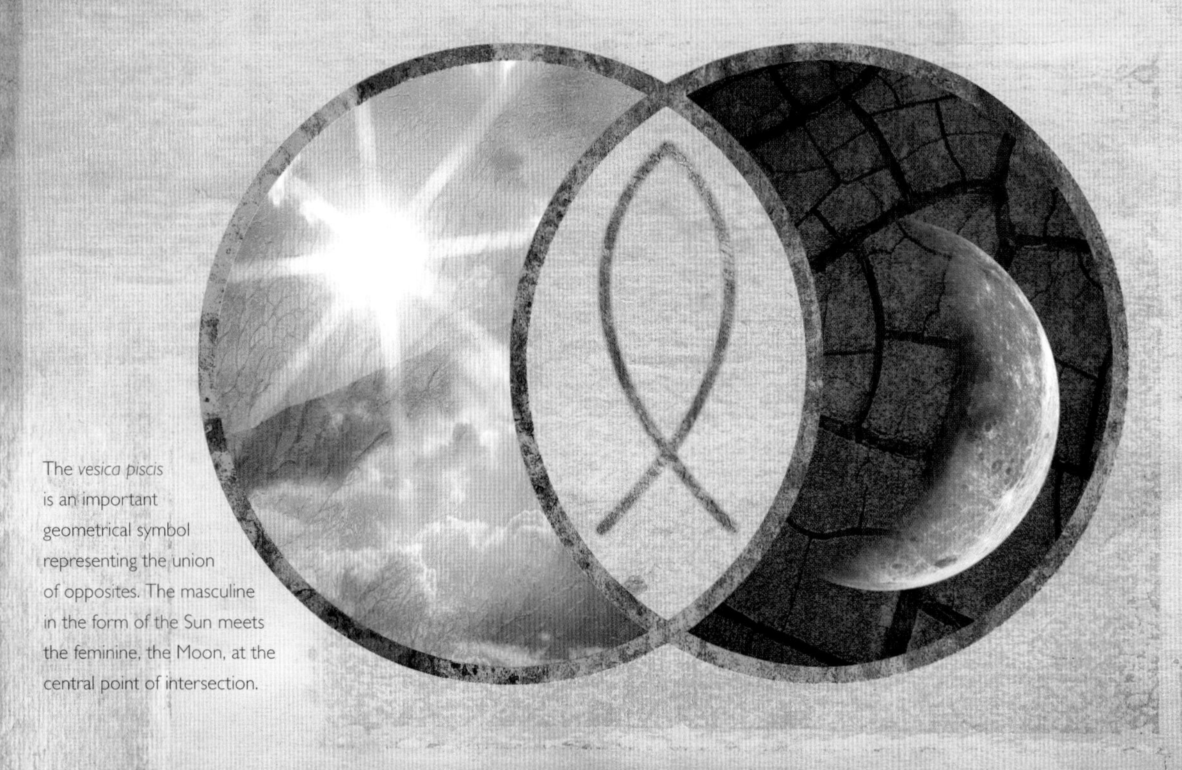

The *vesica piscis* is an important geometrical symbol representing the union of opposites. The masculine in the form of the Sun meets the feminine, the Moon, at the central point of intersection.

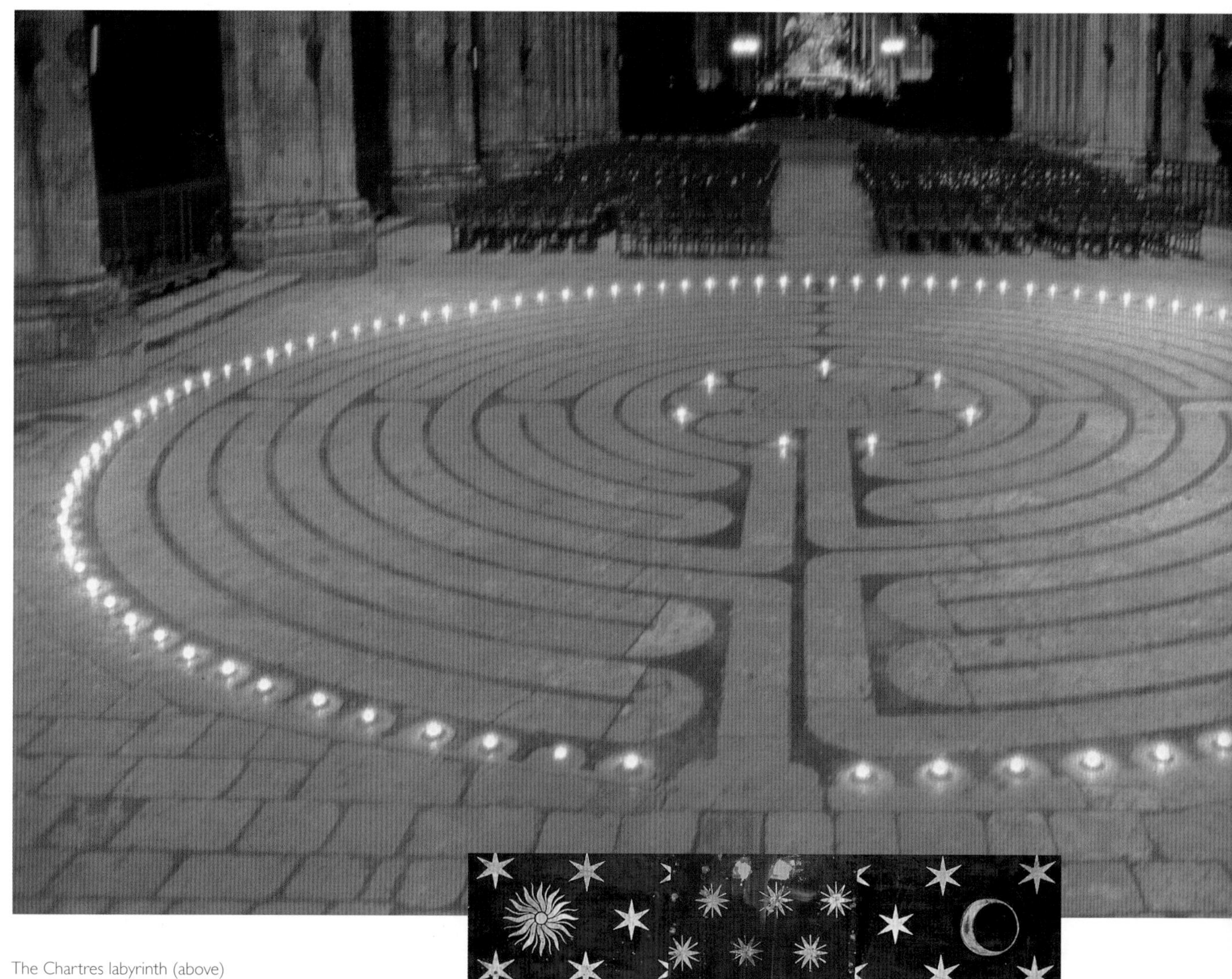

The Chartres labyrinth (above) brought to life by candlelight.

The Sun and Moon in this ceiling fresco (right) illustrate the dialogue of opposites in Chartres Cathedral. The hand shows God's all-pervading influence over the macrocosm.

The well in the crypt of Chartres Cathedral (far right).

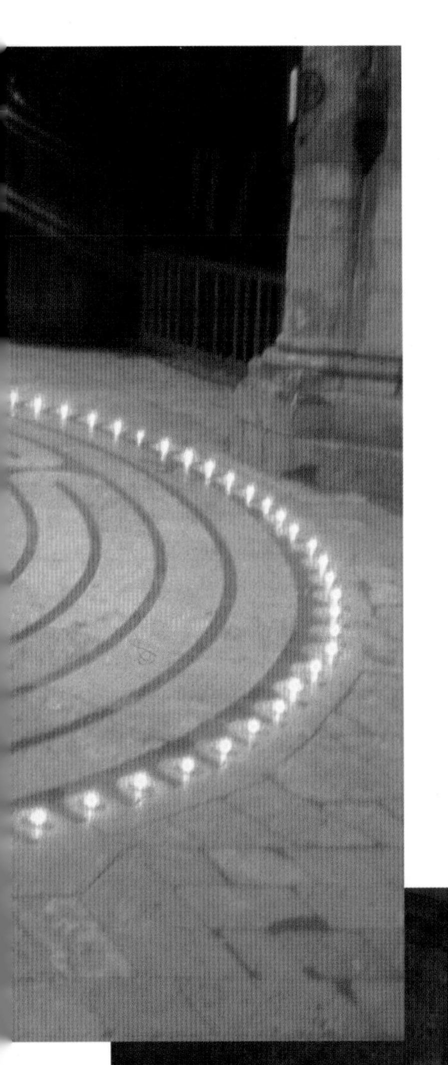

phoenix sculpture. The two forms of celebration, the Christian and the New Age, were held in strong balance at the Chalice Well, where people from both events came to join our group. Together we meditated and danced on the labyrinth and drank the pure spring water.

The next day, when we lifted up the canvas, a circular mandala shape was imprinted on the grass from the rhythmic movement of feet on the labyrinth, like the tracks of animals at a waterhole. What was the purpose behind this quest? Were we simply seeking ordinary water? The pure water of the Chalice Well spring gives us a clue: it is primary water that has never been part of the rain-water cycle, pure and charged with the Earth's energies as it rises up from the depths below. I knew deep down that the labyrinth, through the agency of human movement, works on the interface between spirit and matter, unlocking energy in the earth beneath and in human hearts within. Touched by love in the chamber of the heart, purity begins to flow, giving new life.

Water in the form of rain and of tears was one of the great gifts of the pilgrimage to Chartres in April 2000, the culmination of my journey with the labyrinth. Fifty pilgrims from the United Kingdom, France, and New Zealand walked across muddy fields towards Chartres, the spires of the cathedral rising slowly above the horizon to greet us. We brought with us spring, river, and lake water in bottles from our different home places to give as offerings to the Eure River at the foot of Chartres. Above us rose the mound of the city crowned by the cathedral and, in its crypt, a deep, ancient well. In the pouring rain, I emptied my bottle of water from Chalice Well into the Eure as a fellow pilgrim emptied her bottle of water from its counterpart in New Zealand, Lake Taupo. My prayer was that each pilgrim would receive streams of blessing and grace from our pilgrimage, and that my dryness of heart would end. Later that day, as I reached a turning point on the canvas labyrinth, a fellow pilgrim gave me a long hug. I felt warmed and accepted. Tears came later: my prayer was being answered.

Another great gift of the pilgrimage for me was exploring turnings, whether small as the pathway meets a labrys shape on the labyrinth (see p. 64), or large in the huge U-shaped crypt running the entire length of the cathedral. As I walked along the crypt, deep underneath the cathedral floor, I felt I was making a passage into the earth-body of *Notre Dame de Sous-Terre* (Our Lady Under-the-Earth). I passed her wooden statue and her deep well and, at the apex, where there is a chapel aligned with the Moon's rising, turned to walk down the other side of the U-shape toward the baptismal font. As I walked my body was learning through movement to acknowledge the present moment and what has happened in the past. At the turns, where I felt fully protected by the feminine, I could let go of the past and move into new life.

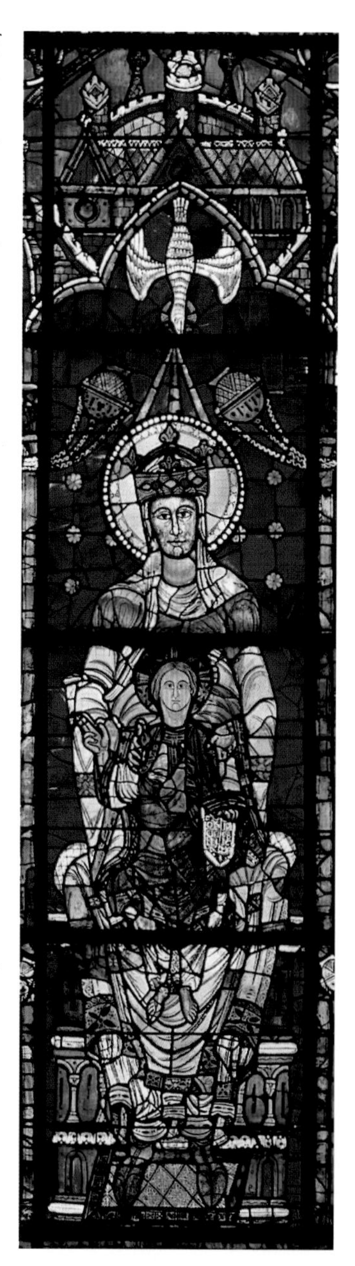

We also trod the U-turn high in the air, when our guide took us up a spiral staircase to the outside of the cathedral. We walked around the sanctuary at the level of the stained-glass windows and underneath the flying buttresses. I looked through a piece of sage-green stained-glass window into the body of the cathedral below, and was awed by the sight of the huge space, green as if submerged beneath the sea and extending as far as the three west portal windows beyond. I felt part of a great transforming power welling up from the depths of the cathedral. As we rounded the northern corner, the whole group broke into a spontaneous song and dance of praise to Mary.

That night I trod the myriad turns on the original labyrinth set into the stone floor of the cathedral by the west door. The group spread evenly around the circumference of the labyrinth, forming a human wall holding the journeys of those within with our presence and with a low humming "O" sound. I felt the labyrinth become a great bowl of moving prayer. I entered and, at the first turn, felt one hand move to palm-down position, the other palm-up, giving me a tentative, new experience of receiving as well as giving, of being as well as doing. I rested with this in the center, my eyes looking up to the beautiful blue light of the three west windows and the rose window above, my bare feet resting on the old stone trodden by so many pilgrims before. As I came out of the labyrinth I felt released into new life, free of pathways and roaming in glorious light.

Toward the end of the pilgrimage I received another gift, that of reconnection. During the pilgrimage we explored different layers of time through Greek, medieval, and modern Circle Dance, and through stories told by a gifted storyteller. I felt each dance and story awakened a different layer of my memory. But it was when I stood in front of the stained-glass window of *Notre-Dame de la Belle Verrière* (left), showing Mary in majesty enthroned with Jesus on her lap, that my memory surprised me with a new connection. Her robe is an almond-shape of blue, the central shape of the *vesica piscis* I knew from Glastonbury. This blue was also the color of the bluebells I used to pick in May as a child and take to school to put on the little classroom altar honoring Mary. Standing underneath the soft light of the window, I felt I could have been standing there with a bunch of bluebells in my hand, being welcomed into the warmth of the house of Mary.

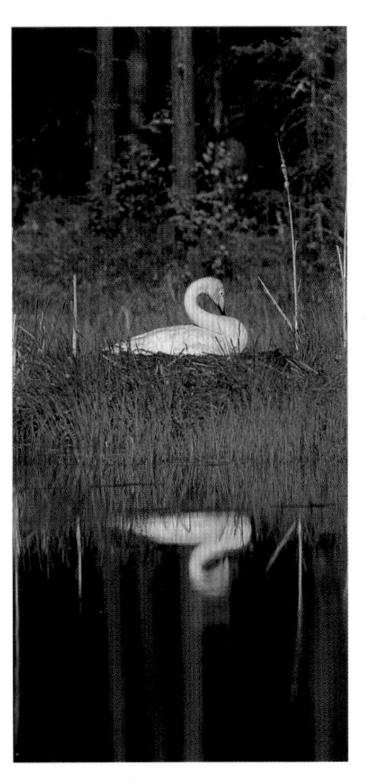

I could leave behind the hurt I had felt as a young mother, and the feeling of exclusion as a woman from the Church. Reconciliation graced my heart, the center space of the *vesica piscis*. The rose of love could now grow.

Each individual pilgrim followed her own path, and her own story on the pilgrimage. Our group was vibrant with life as we ate, talked, laughed, and sang together. On the last day I asked for all the names of places visited over the three-year pilgrimage to be read out from the memory thread (see pp. 12–13). I then cut the thread as a sign that we had made our passage into the new millennium with the labyrinth and that the pilgrimage was complete.

As we started our journey home, walking down the hill and crossing the Eure River, my gaze fell upon a swan sleeping in a fork between the waters. White, beautiful, and at rest, it reminded me of Mary in her purity and grace. It was a symbol of life, bringing with it the new dawn of the day. The pilgrimage had ended, but my journey with the labyrinth would continue to unfold.

Afoot and lighthearted I take to the open road
Healthy, free, the world before me
The long brown path before me leading wherever I choose.
Walt Whitman

I

Labyrinths: a universal symbol

This book celebrates the labyrinth and the inspiration it has given people from ancient times to the present day. It is intended as a starting point for your own exploration, from which you can develop your personal path on the labyrinth. For this purpose I draw on my experience of working with different designs, in particular the one on the floor of Chartres Cathedral in France.

Our ancestors used the labyrinth shape through the ages and left behind a legacy of labyrinth artifacts that continue to capture our imaginations today. The beauty of this shape lies in its universal appeal, for it is not attached to any one faith or tradition, so each person who follows its path can draw from it what he or she needs. The labyrinth is a means of meditation offering us space to listen to ourselves. It can be a slow and contemplative experience or fast and energizing; it can help us shed layers of emotion and unravel a problem; or it can stimulate the mind and offer inspiration. The physical movement toward the labyrinth's center is echoed by an inward movement to the deep center inside each of us, where we are whole and intact even if we are ill or suffering. The path of the labyrinth, therefore—takes us on an inner journey of healing toward personal well-being and newness of spirit.

Chapter One will begin your journey with the labyrinth by tracing it across millennia in nature, myth, and history. Chapter Two examines ways in which you can prepare yourself and others to tread the labyrinth, while Chapter Three explores your experience on its path. You can discover ways to ground yourself and fellow pilgrims when you leave the labyrinth in Chapter Four, and learn how to make your own labyrinth in Chapter Five—from simple line drawings to more ambitious projects using stones, canvas, or sand.

Labyrinths and mazes

Although labyrinths and mazes can be found all over the world, many have been neglected, destroyed, or simply forgotten over time. Recently they have begun to grip our imaginations once more, and original

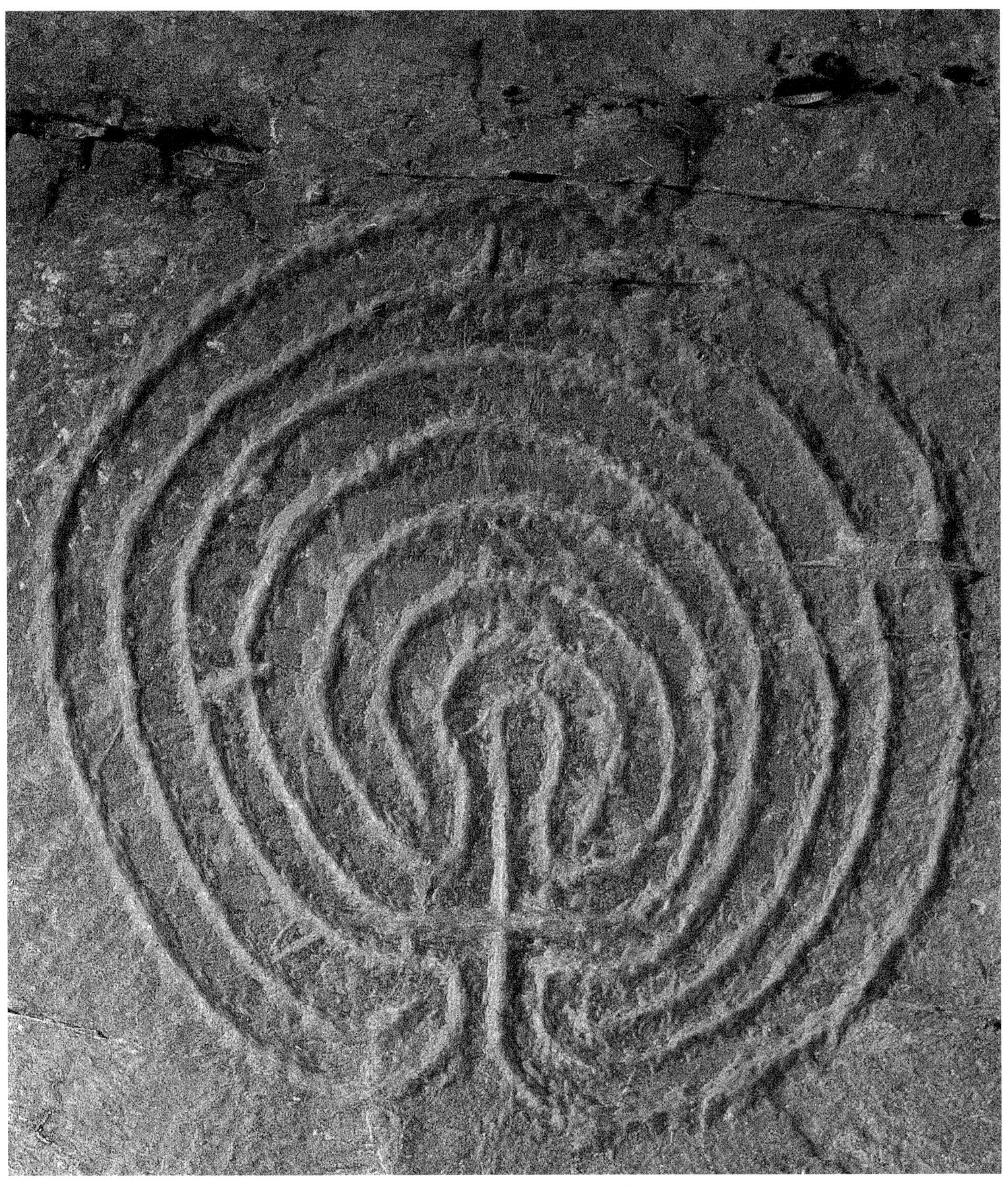

One of two rock carvings at Rocky Valley, Tintagel in Cornwall, England, with coins pushed into the rock face above. Probably 18th century, although it may date from as early as the Bronze Age.

designs are now being restored and replicas of them made across the globe. Modern innovative designs are proving just as popular. Traditionally the words "labyrinth" and "maze" were used interchangeably, but they have since assumed quite different meanings: labyrinths are unicursal with only one pathway, which twists and turns to a central goal, while mazes are multicursal with one correct path leading to the center hidden amongst numerous dead ends and junctions. However, this distinction is a modern one, so you may find a number of older English turf labyrinths with the name "Maze" or "Mizmaze."

Although walkers on a labyrinth have to give their full attention to following the path, they will not face any decisions to turn left or right; instead, the left side of the brain governing actions associated with the right side of the body—verbal, rational, logical, linear, abstract—can rest and the right side of the brain controlling responses attributed to the left side of the body—nonverbal, nonrational, intuitive, synthetic, concrete—can be exercised. Western society encourages a dominance of left-brain work, which interferes with the delicate balance between the two hemispheres of the brain. Treading labyrinths can help to correct this imbalance.

Conversely, mazes encourage left-brain activity as the walker has to make conscious decisions to turn one way or another. These puzzles are a development of the original unicursal labyrinth and became popular in the 15th century in French and Italian Renaissance gardens. They were used for recreation and romantic dalliance. Mazes continue to be popular today, which is perhaps a reflection of our need to find order in our modern, often chaotic society. A journey in a maze, with its outward focus and spirit of adventure, is very different from one in a labyrinth where the focus is inward and sometimes meditative. For this reason we will now leave the maze to explore the unicursal path of the labyrinth.

Evoking the past; evoking nature

When we see a picture of a labyrinth we are instantly fascinated. Its twists and turns mirror inner body design; the coiling surface of the brain, the labyrinth of the inner ear, the loops of the small intestine. In effect, if you look at a labyrinth, you can see in it a reflection of your inner landscape. Similarly, the Theseus and Ariadne story often associated with the labyrinth (see p. 32) connects us with Ariadne's thread twining through the labyrinth to the center. Perhaps this stirs our subconscious and takes us back to the womb, when we were attached to the life-giving umbilical cord.

We can also see the shape of the labyrinth all around us in the spiraling and turnings of nature: in the swirl of a thumbprint, in water rippling outwards, in spiders' webs, in the uncoiling of a fern. From these images we can recognize the journey of growth and becoming, curling and circling outward and inward like the labyrinth. For this reason we follow a familiar path on the labyrinth, as if we were returning to the source of life itself.

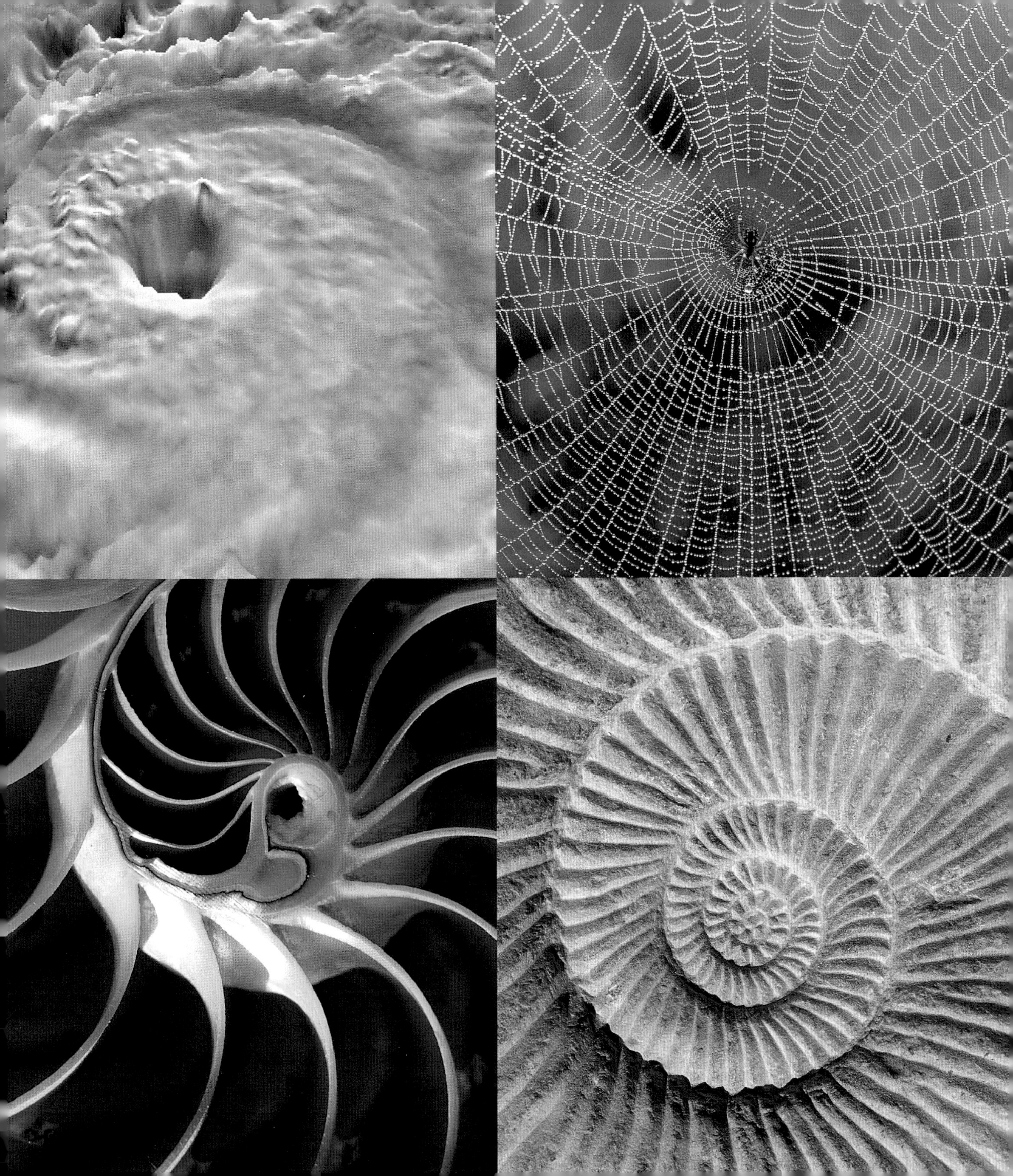

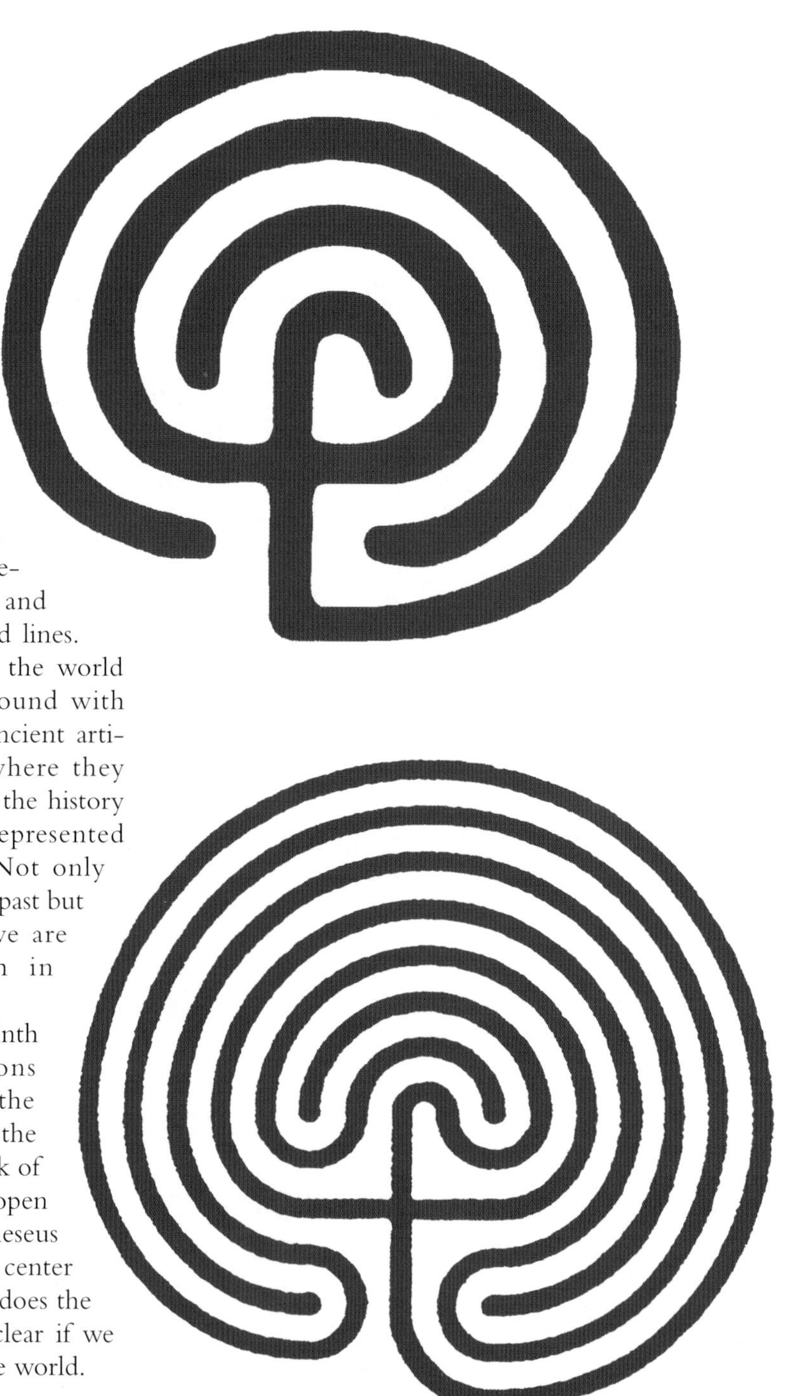

One path, many designs

The origins of unicursal labyrinths stretch back in time over thousands of years. The earliest and simplest examples—perhaps used for ritual purposes—are thought to date from around 2500 B.C. This labyrinth design is the three-circuit labyrinth (top right) constructed around two crossed lines at the central axis.

The classical labyrinth design (bottom right) is an extension of this simple three-circuit labyrinth and has seven circuits and eight walls around the central two crossed lines. The classical labyrinth is found all over the world traced on rock, marked out on the ground with stones, carved into turf and decorating ancient artifacts. If we study these designs and where they are found we can begin to piece together the history of the labyrinth, what it might have represented and how it was used over millennia. Not only is this fascinating in terms of decoding the past but it also sheds light on why and how we are moved to use the labyrinth afresh in the 21st century.

The central space of the classical labyrinth has evolved into three permutations over time: crossed lines at the center (the destination is the small quarter space in the top right-hand corner, resembling the hook of a walking stick or shepherd's crook); an open center space, containing a depiction of Theseus and the Minotaur; and an open and empty center space. As the center space changes, so too does the role of the labyrinth. This will become clear if we examine specific examples from all over the world.

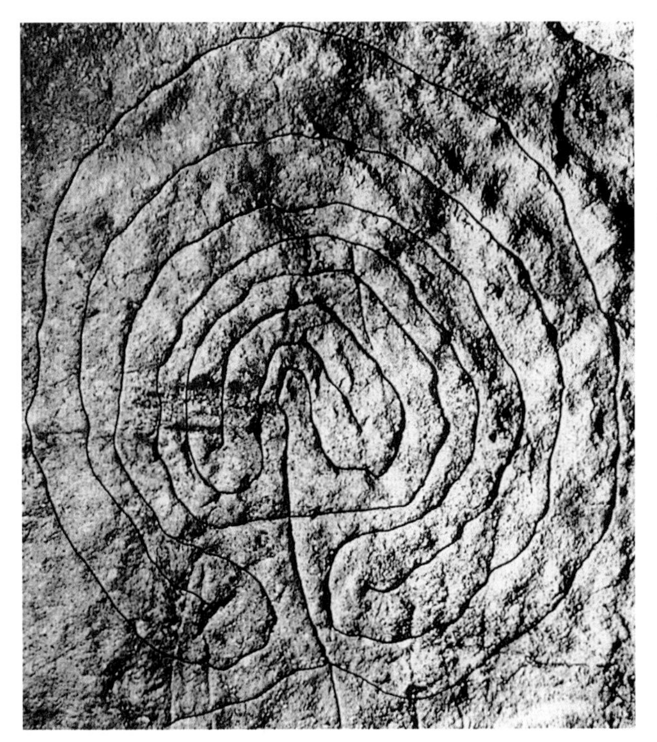

Pathway for rites of passage

The classical design with a central cross can be found on artifacts belonging to many different cultures across the world. The oldest existing example to date is a labyrinth carved into the rock of a Neolithic chambered tomb in Luzzanas, Sardinia (see left), dating from 2500–2000 B.C. Although the labyrinth may have been added later as graffiti, its presence in the tomb gives us a clue about the labyrinth's connection with the rituals of life and death: group ceremonial dancing and movement could have traced the passage back to the Earth Mother at death and through the gateway of the tomb.

The cross at the center of this basic labyrinth seems to suggest the four directions, north, south, east, and west, honored in the Native American tradition. Indeed, labyrinths believed to date from the 12th century have been found carved into rock faces in Hopi reservations in northern Arizona. The Hopi labyrinth is a symbol of Emergence, or birth and creation, and is known as Mother Earth. It appears in two forms, the first, *Tápu'at*, meaning Mother and Child, whose squared pathway lines simultaneously suggest the baby curled in the womb and the newborn infant cradled in loving arms. The straight line at the entrance/exit to the labyrinth represents both the umbilical cord and the birth canal. The meaning of the second elongated and rounded version is slightly different: it symbolizes the Sun Father, the giver of life, and its pathway the journey through life. This version also denotes the concentric boundaries of territories that were claimed by the Hopi.

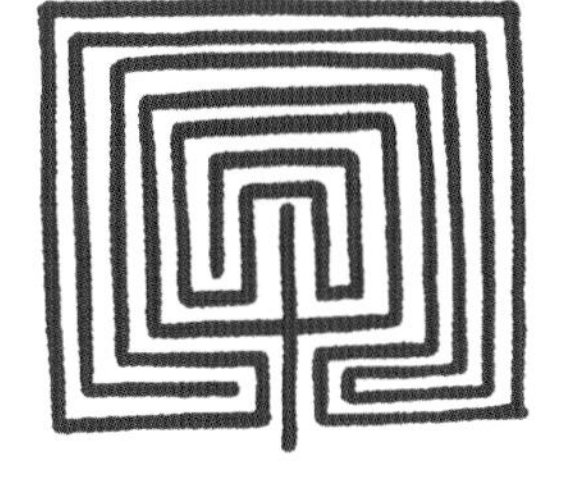

The labyrinth carved into a Neolithic tomb at Luzzanas in Sardinia (above) may have been made as early as 2500 B.C. Measuring about 12 inches (30 cm.) in diameter, it is the oldest recorded labyrinth in the world. The Labyrinth was thought to be a map to help the soul through the underworld after death.

The two labyrinths (right) are variations on the Hopi symbol of Emergence and are closely equated with the themes of rebirth and regeneration.

Labyrinths for fun

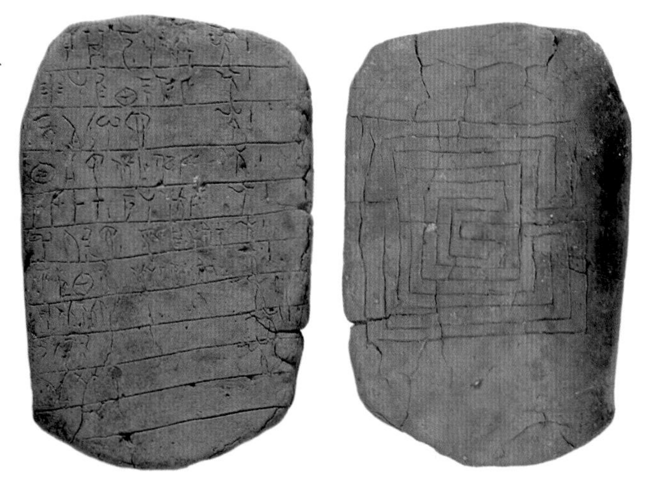

An inscribed clay tablet from the Mycenaean palace of Pylos in southern Greece (right) dates from 1200 B.C. and shows a variant of the round labyrinth design: the pathways are pulled into a square shape with its corners resting on diagonal axes that radiate from the center space. This shape appears frequently in later Roman labyrinth designs. The tablet is slightly larger than the average man's hand and is of particular interest as the top of the tablet was used to record the delivery of goats. The inclusion of the labyrinth on the other side suggests that it was part of ordinary life—perhaps the labyrinth was a game like tick-tack-toe; or perhaps it was simply a doodle, which could be traced with the finger or eye to soothe or focus the mind.

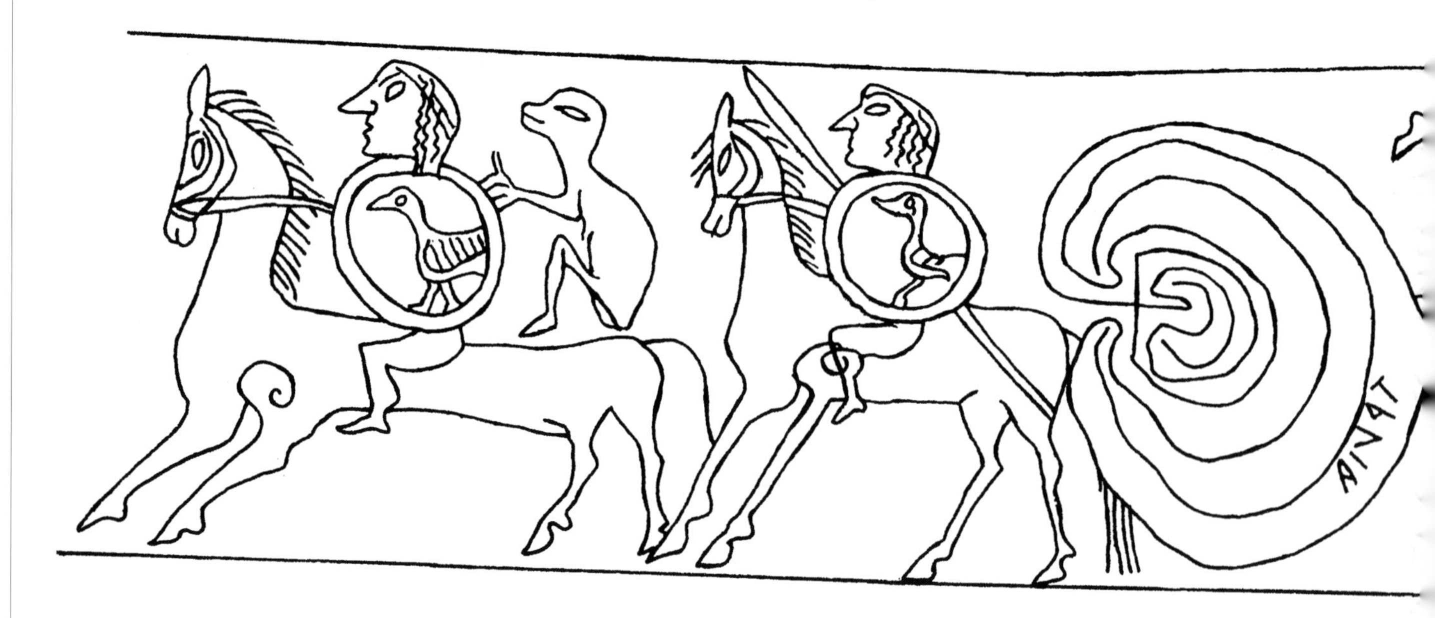

The walled city of Troy

An Etruscan wine jar found at Tragliatella, Italy, dating from the late 7th century B.C., shows a circular labyrinth with the word *Truia*, or Troy, written on a pathway (below left). There are also some important pictorial additions on either side of the design. Two horses, mounted by rider-warriors brandishing shields and spears, stride away from the mouth of the labyrinth. Behind the labyrinth two men mount two women in intercourse. A bardic man wrapped in his tunic stands to the right with his arm gesturing toward them. Perhaps he is telling Homer's story of the fall of the fortified city of Troy, which was besieged by the Greeks for ten years. Helen, wife of the Greek King Menelaus, was abducted by Paris and taken to Troy. In this depiction the labyrinth is equated with Troy, the walled city guarding the beautiful woman, Helen, at its center. Sexual union or rape (the couples) and bloody warfare (the warriors) are the bones of the story. The inviolable fortress was eventually penetrated by trickery: the Greeks hid inside a wooden horse, which was dragged by the unsuspecting Trojans inside the city walls. Later they emerged and razed the city to the ground.

This theme of the labyrinth as a besieged city is also found on a different continent, in India, in a manuscript dating from around A.D. 1045 telling the Ramayana epic. The labyrinth represents the Ravana fortress, where the beautiful Sita was taken by the wicked demon Ravana after he had snatched her from her husband, Rama. With the help of some monkeys, Rama eventually rescued her.

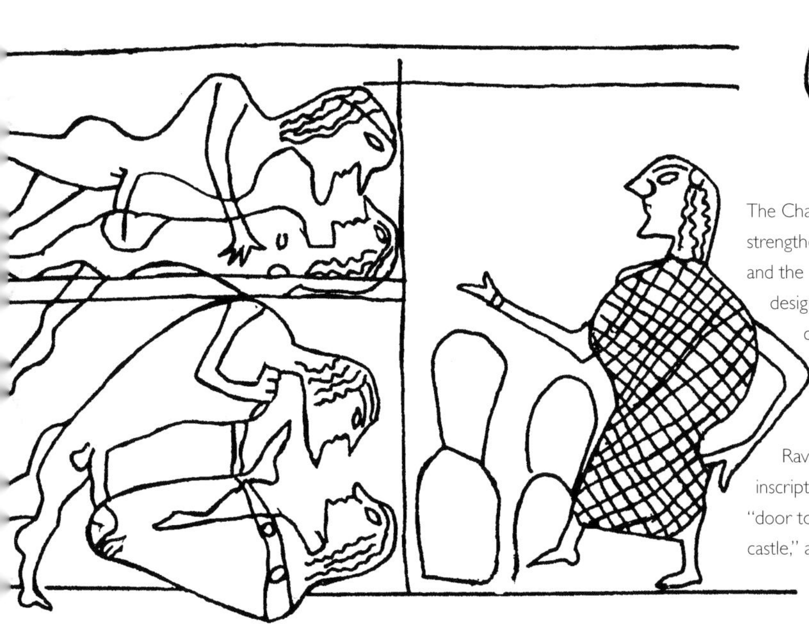

The Chakra-vyuha yantra (above) strengthens the link between birth and the labyrinth. This yantra was designed to help the unborn child find its way out of the labyrinthine uterus, thereby easing birth. It is, curiously, an inverted copy of the Ravana labyrinth (right). The inscription at the entrance reads "door to the road leading to the castle," and at the center "castle."

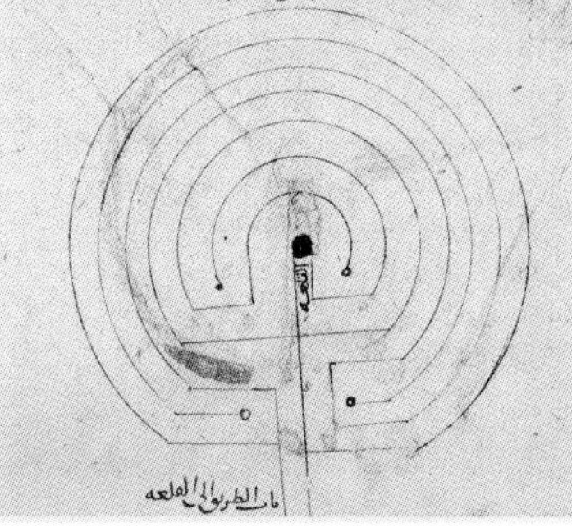

Trapping evil spirits

The Tragliatella wine jar is the first evidence of linking Troy to the labyrinth. This later became a tradition in Sweden, Germany, Finland, and Denmark, and a number of outdoor labyrinths with names such as Troyaburg, Trojienborg, or Trojborg can still be seen in these countries today. Their pathways are defined by stones arranged on the ground and are large enough to walk on. Further south, turf mazes were also popular, although many have since been lost or destroyed. These were made by cutting away the surface soil and grass to form indented walls, leaving

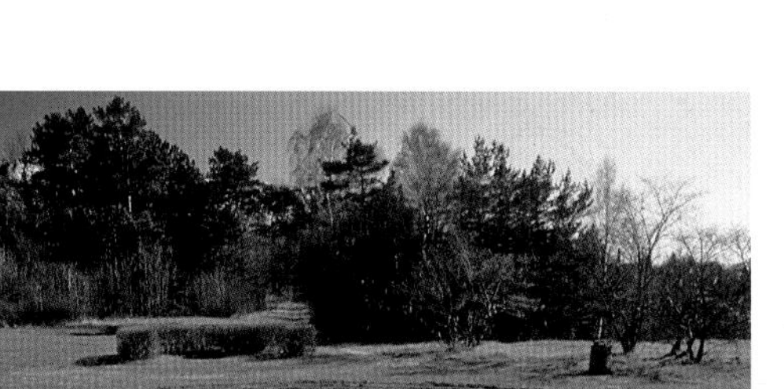

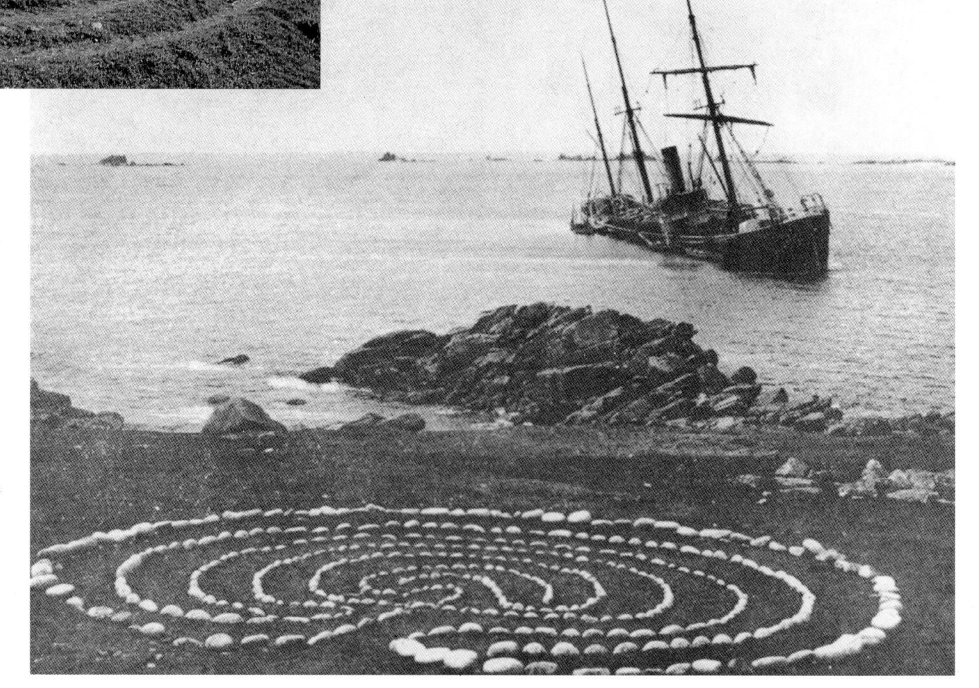

One spectacular example that was probably constructed in the 13th century can be found at Visby on the island of Gotland in Sweden (above). Although its paths are cut into turf, stones are also used to line them. It lies near the sea and was walked by fishermen to help them entrap bad weather before fishing expeditions.

Troy Town on St. Agnes, Scilly Isles (right), is thought to have been built by a lighthouse keeper in 1729. The shipwreck behind the stone paths is a sober reminder of the merciless sea and the justifiable fears and superstitions of local fishermen.

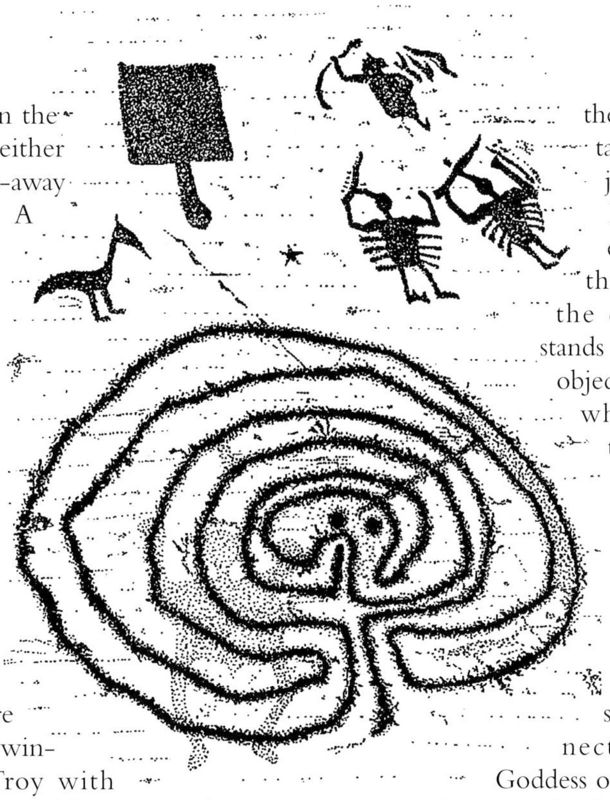

grassy ridges. Depending on the design people would tread either on the grass or on the cut-away earth to reach the center. A number of turf labyrinths have survived in Great Britain and kept their Troy-related names, such as the City of Troy, Troy-town, the Walls of Troy, and the Welsh turf labyrinth, Caerdroia.

The Troy labyrinths were used as a protection against many evils, such as bad weather, mischievous spirits, and trolls. Sometimes they were associated with the sport of winning maidens, linking Troy with Helen, the personification of beauty, and echoing fairy tales of valiant knights rescuing maidens from tower prisons. Local girls would stand at the center of the labyrinth while boys sped in to try to reach and claim them first.

Fertility and the crane

There are at least five early Iron Age labyrinths (circa 750–500 B.C.) carved into the rock face at Naquane, Val Camonica, in northern Italy (above), and one in particular adds a new element to the design. Ususally the walls of the labyrinth contain the pilgrim on his or her journey to the center, but here the line of the design etched into the rock traces the actual pathway. Outside the circuits of this labyrinth stands a long-necked bird, a square object, and three humans holding what could be sticks above their heads. All three figures have feather-like extensions jutting out from their ribs. The bird could be a crane and the humans dancers imitating its mating display of raised wings and calling sounds. This may have connected them to the Mother Goddess of fertility, new life and compassion, who is often associated with the crane. A Crane Dance called *Geranos* is also linked to the myth of Theseus and the Minotaur, which is a celebration of sexual potency and fertility. Theseus and Ariadne are said to have danced it when they arrived at the island of Naxos after fleeing Crete. A Greek form of *Geranos* exists today in Circle Dance. It is called *Tsakonikos* (see pp. 72–73) and is performed in snaking lines of dancers. The right thumb is held in the left hand of the next dancer to highlight its sexual significance.

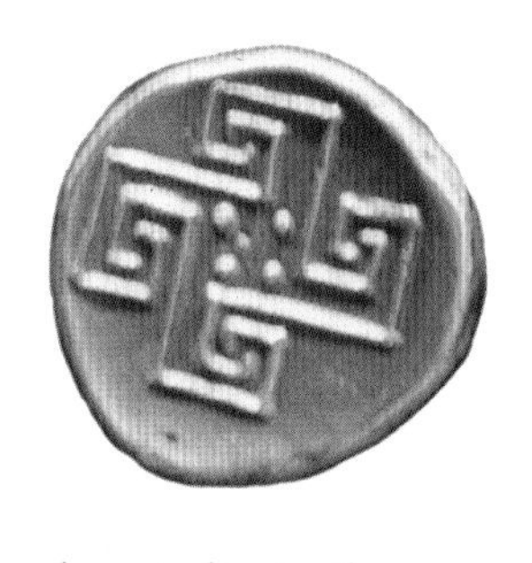

The myth of Theseus, Ariadne, and the Minotaur became the central story connected with the labyrinth in Europe, and illustrates a new departure in labyrinth folklore: before, the woman—represented by the beautiful Helen—was waiting to be saved at the heart of an impregnable fortress; now, the woman—in the form of the compassionate Ariadne—holds the cord of life so the man can find his way after his heroic ordeal. When the site of the palace of Knossos was excavated by Arthur Evans in the early 20th century, no labyrinth was found, although the construction of the palace itself was labyrinthine and not dissimilar to a temple structure built by King Amenamhet III in Fayum, Egypt, around 1800 B.C. However, many Cretan coins inscribed with a variety of labyrinths have been found at Knossos, which indicate the labyrinth's cultural significance and how closely it was linked to Cretan identity. The three examples (above and below left) date from 425–67 B.C. We can begin to appreciate the impact of the legend of Theseus and the Minotaur on the rest of world if we examine the next development in labyrinth design.

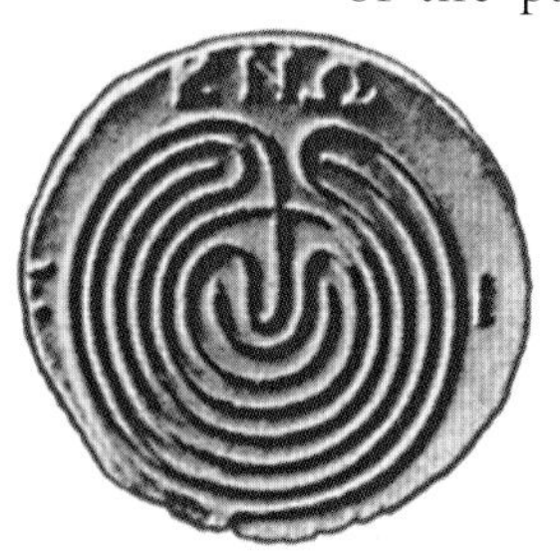

Theseus and the Minotaur

The labyrinth has long been associated with Knossos, for according to legend the palace of Knossos stood over the great labyrinth that was constructed by the inventor Daedalus to house the Minotaur, half-man, half-beast. The Minotaur was the monster offspring of Queen Pasiphae and a white sacrificial bull, and the labyrinth was intended to keep him out of sight.

Every nine years the Minotaur was fed tribute victims from Athens in requital for the death of King Minos' son, Androgeus. Seven young men and seven young women were chosen for the fateful voyage to Crete. One year, Theseus, son of King Aegeus of Athens, volunteered to go. He promised his father that if he succeeded in killing the Minotaur he would, when he sailed back to Athens, change the ship's sail from black to white.

They sailed to Crete and, upon arrival, Ariadne, daughter of King Minos, fell in love with Theseus. She vowed to help Theseus provided he took her away with him if he survived. She gave him a ball of gold thread to unravel behind him as he went into the labyrinth so that, if he succeeded in killing the Minotaur, he would be able to wind up the thread and find his way out. It is true that if the labyrinth were unicursal, as the designs on the coins show, then Theseus should have been able to find his way out unassisted. Perhaps we have to interpret the story on a symbolic level: underground in the dark, womb-like labyrinth the hero needs to hold the illuminating thread of the feminine to find his way from death to new life.

Theseus entered the labyrinth, met the Minotaur at the center and killed him. He then reeled in the thread, found his way out of the labyrinth and escaped from Crete with Ariadne. On the island of Naxos they celebrated their escape and union by dancing *Geranos*, the Crane Dance.

Afterwards, Theseus forgot his two promises: first, he deserted Ariadne on the island and sailed away without her; and second, he forgot to put up the white sail for his return journey. As he approached Athens his father, looking out from the cliffs, saw the black sail and threw himself into the sea in despair. The sea bears his name to this day—the Aegean. Theseus was hailed as the new king, his heart heavy with grief.

Theseus victorious in the center

The Roman Empire yields many examples of mosaic pavement labyrinths, dating from circa 165 B.C. to A.D. 400. The classical labyrinth is developed by opening up the central space and pushing the four axes, north, south, east, and west, outward to act as the boundaries of four quarters, each one containing a classical labyrinth. The four labyrinths are connected and follow in systematic order to the center goal. They are usually too small to be walked so may have served a decorative or protective function. Often the center contains a picture of Theseus—either in full or just his helmeted head—and the Minotaur. The first century A.D. mosaic (below left) found at Via Cadolini, Cremona, in Italy is a good example of such a labyrinth. Here Theseus is lunging at the Minotaur, who is crouching before him subjugated. The outer walls of the labyrinth are crenellated and each corner has a fortification tower, which emphasizes the difficulty of Theseus' heroic task: he had to penetrate the labyrinth domain before he could kill the monster within.

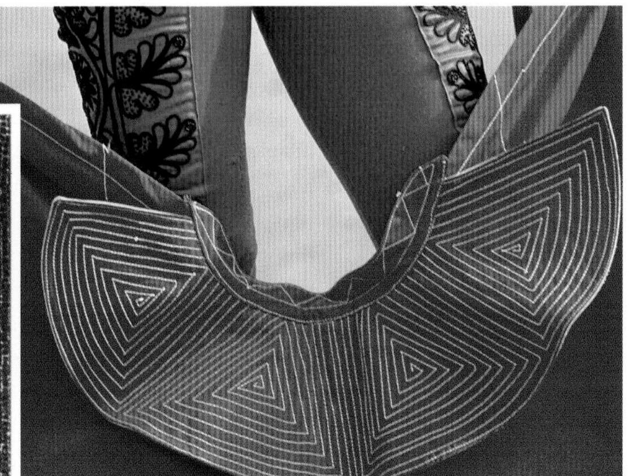

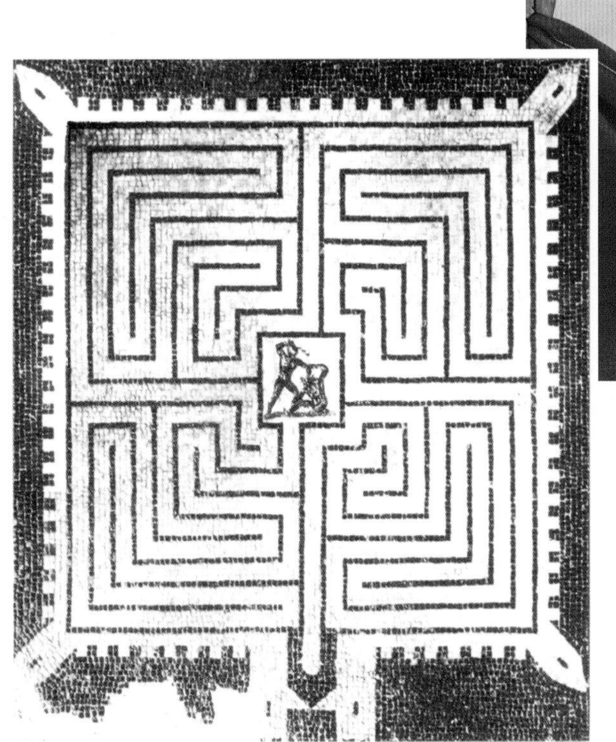

The tradition of bullfighting can be linked to the legend of Theseus and the Minotaur. In Spain the bull is often chased through the streets of the town before entering the bullring to meet the matador. The race through the town can be likened to the journey through the labyrinth and the sacrifice in the bullring to the slaying of the Minotaur at the center.

An open, empty center

The labyrinth developed significantly in the Middle Ages and found its way into European Christian cathedrals. The pathways increased from seven to eleven in number, and the north, south, east, and west axes were broken at different places. The pathway to the center swung apparently at random from one quarter to the next, with the effect of disorientating the treader. These labyrinths were often very large and intended to be walked. The center was open without an image of any kind, which points to a shift in emphasis from the stranded woman or fighting hero at the center to a new space of possibility, where the Christian story of salvation could be experienced.

As the Church became increasingly powerful in the Middle Ages, it sought to control or erase supposedly nonChristian rituals. Although the labyrinth was essentially a pagan symbol, the Church found it easy to assimilate it into Christian iconography: with its single path to the center it was a perfect illustration of the single path to salvation. For this reason the labyrinth was left to flourish. For example, the turf Mizmaze at Breamore, near Salisbury, England, is reputed to have been cut by medieval monks, who used it as a penitential pathway to open the way to salvation.

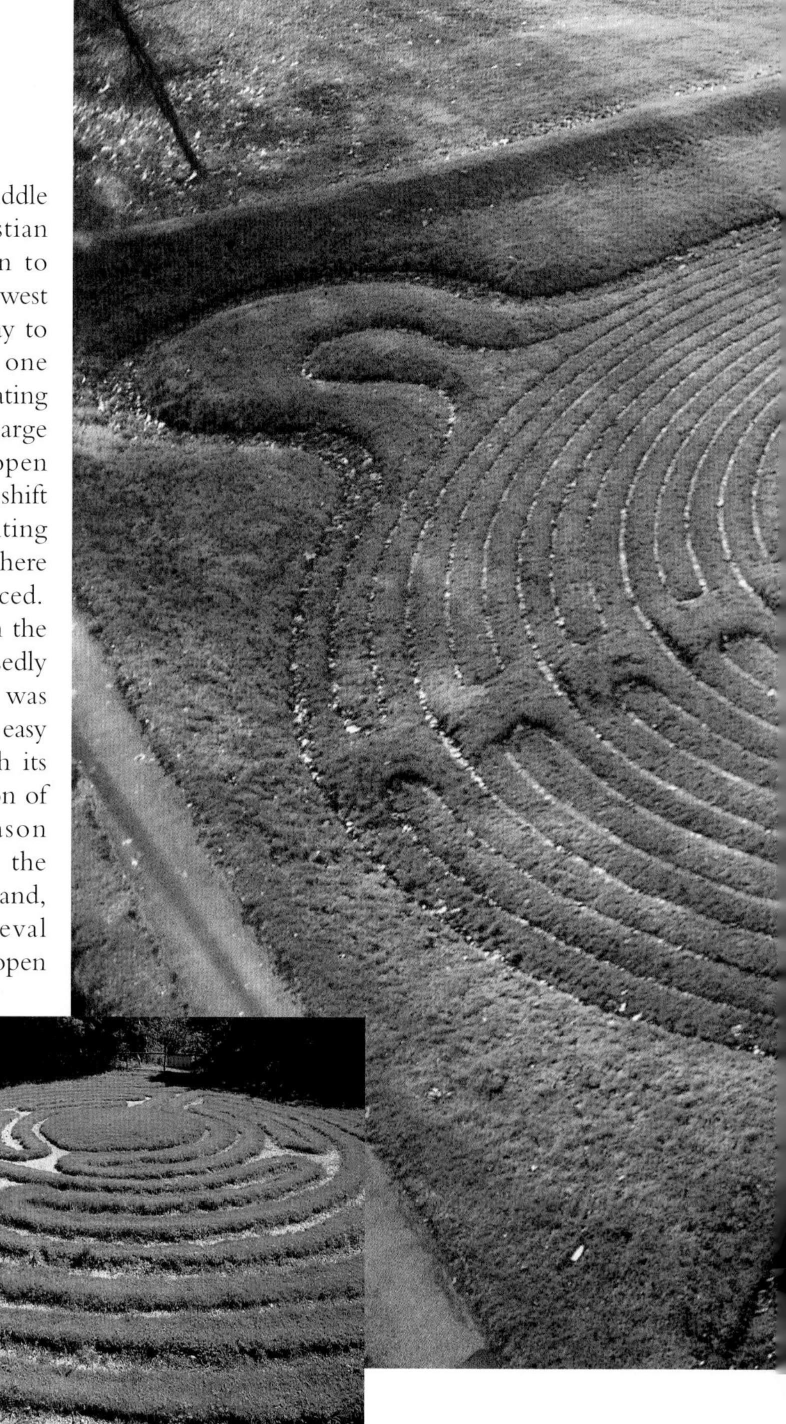

Hidden in a woodland clearing, the medieval Mizmaze at Breamore (right) provides an atmospheric setting for labyrinth pilgrims.

Many ancient labyrinthine rituals survived until quite recently. A record of 1859 describes young men racing through the now 300-year-old turf labyrinth at Saffron Walden in England (far right) to claim girls at the center.

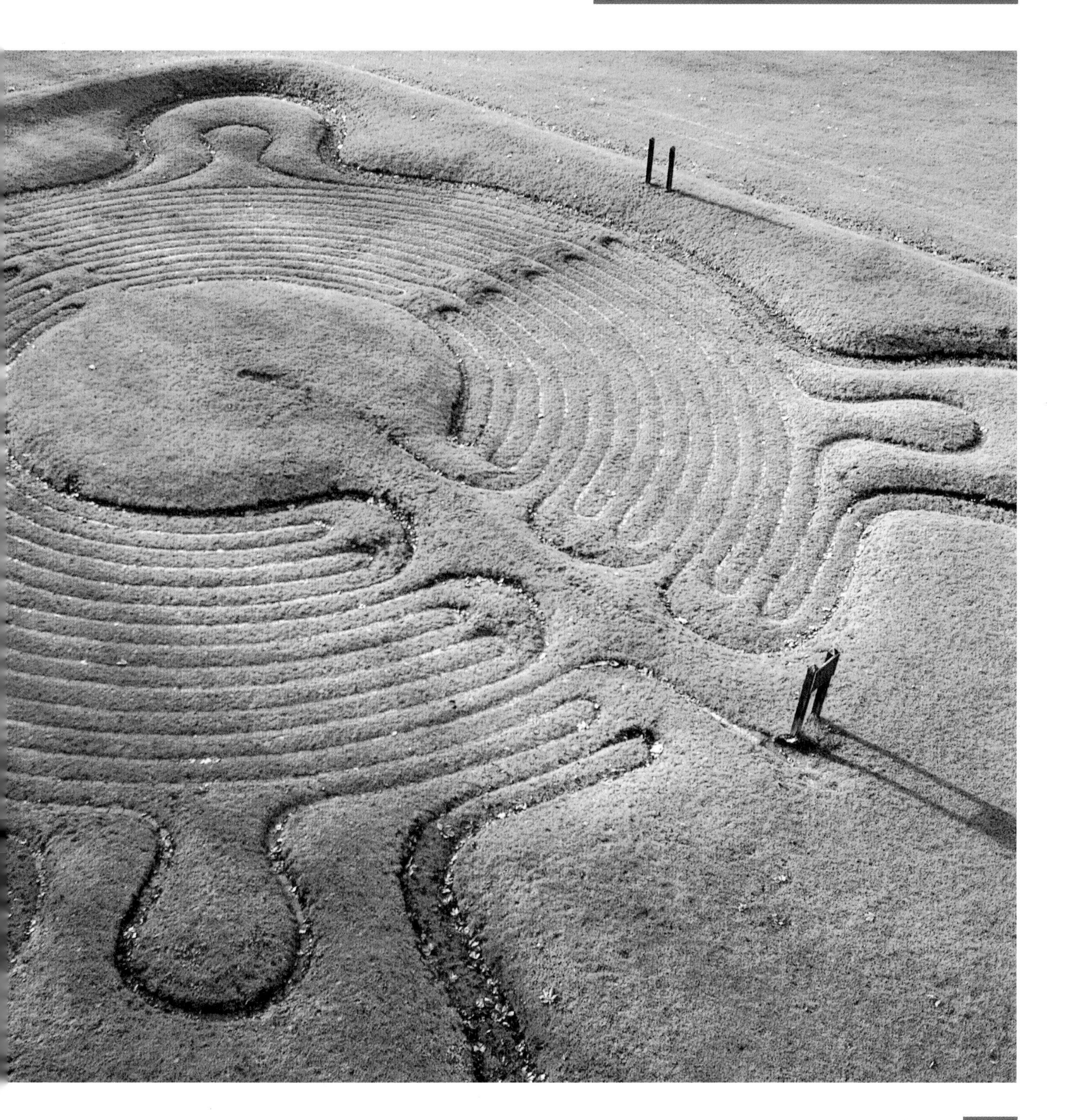

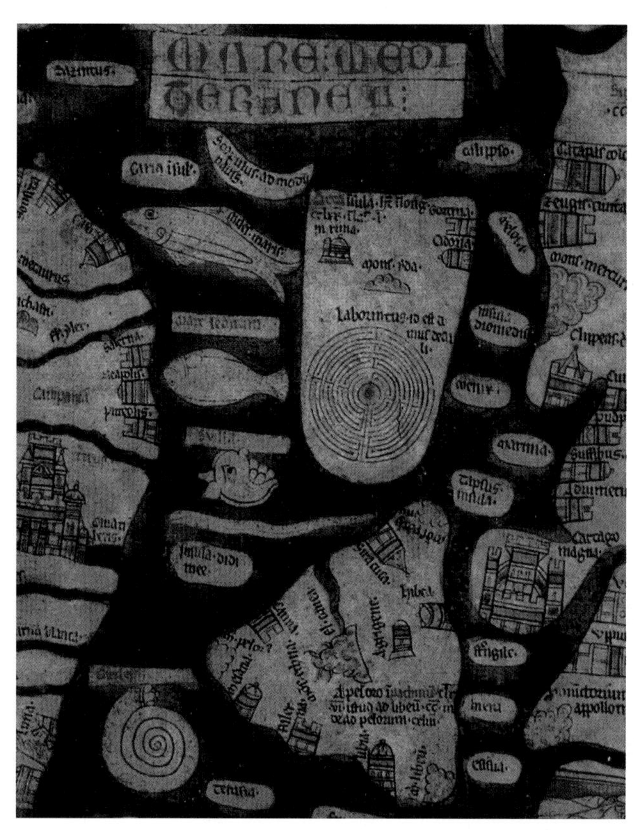

The Mappa Mundi (left), kept in Hereford Cathedral, England, was drawn between 1276 and 1283 in Lincoln, England. It illustrates the extent of the known world at this time, including the seven wonders of the world. Jerusalem lies at the center of the world.

This fragment shows an eleven-circuit labyrinth dominating the island of Crete. It is the same as the design found in Chartres, only the lunations, or teeth, around the circumference are absent, as is the central rose. Fabulous fish and mermaids play alongside in the sea.

Womb of hope

Using the labyrinth as a pathway home to a place of peace or as a form of pilgrimage is also echoed in the design often found on woven baskets made by the Tohono O'odham and Pima tribes of southern Arizona. The design combines the classical labyrinth with an open center. At the entrance to the labyrinth stands an upright man, ready to begin his journey. According to legend, he is Iitoi. Although he saved his people from their wicked ways, some of them turned against him and killed him. His spirit fled to the mountain Baboquivari, where it still lives today. The central space of the labyrinth represents the mountain, the twisting paths his flight.

With the open, empty center the interaction between the masculine and the feminine seems to disappear: there is no Helen figure to rescue from the central walled city of the labyrinth, nor is there an Ariadne to guide the hero on his journey. Yet the feminine influence in the labyrinth has not diminished; instead, like the Hopi labyrinth (see p. 27), it is embodied in the labyrinth itself: what was a walled city to escape from is now a womb of hope and new life to be fertilized by the person who journeys to the center. Just as Iitoi found new life when his spirit fled to Baboquivari, so too can we find a new beginning for ourselves at the heart of the labyrinth.

Path to salvation

The Pima legend is similar to the story of Christ, who saved his people from everlasting death when he died on a cross and rose to new life. His earthly journey ended in Jerusalem, which became a center of pilgrimage for medieval Christians. But the journey there was hazardous, so many pilgrims went to European cathedrals possessing holy relics. Chartres Cathedral in France keeps a relic that is supposed to be part of the Virgin Mary's veil. It is also home to a large labyrinth, which is set in the floor by the west door. Its path became a short form of pilgrimage, and arriving at the center of the labyrinth symbolized arriving at Jerusalem. For this reason it is sometimes called *Le chemin de Jerusalem*, or The Jerusalem Road, also hinting at the New Jerusalem described in the Bible, when all of creation is renewed through Christ.

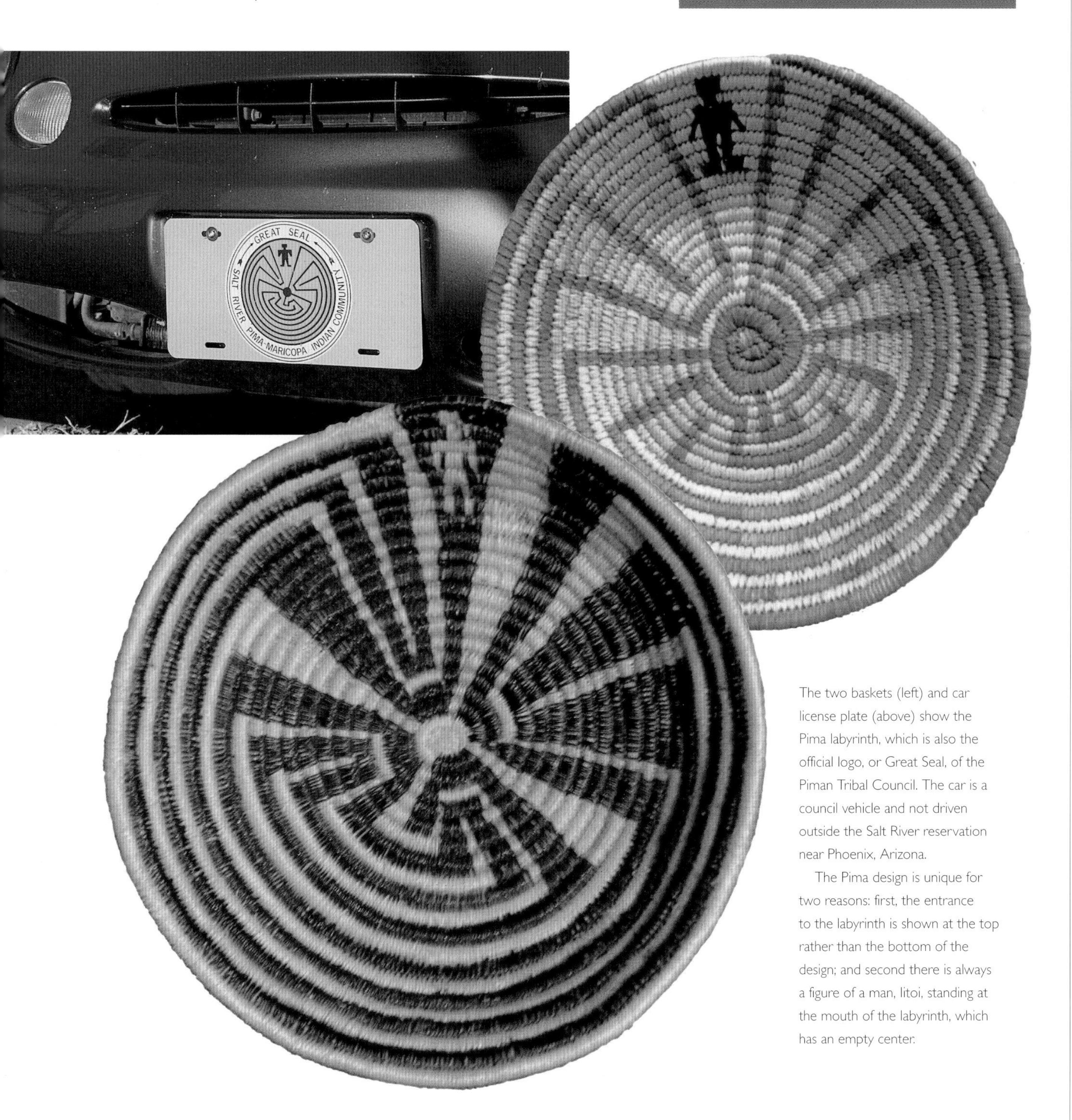

The two baskets (left) and car license plate (above) show the Pima labyrinth, which is also the official logo, or Great Seal, of the Piman Tribal Council. The car is a council vehicle and not driven outside the Salt River reservation near Phoenix, Arizona.

The Pima design is unique for two reasons: first, the entrance to the labyrinth is shown at the top rather than the bottom of the design; and second there is always a figure of a man, Iitoi, standing at the mouth of the labyrinth, which has an empty center.

The petaled center

This central hope of salvation is expressed in the Chartres labyrinth by something new: six flower petals loop around the inner, open space so that the center represents the flowering of energy. This flower form is repeated in the mandala of light in the rose window, situated directly above the labyrinth. The center of the labyrinth and the rose above represent the feminine, embodied by Mary, Mother of Christ in the Christian faith. In the images of flower and path, the masculine and feminine traditions are united: pilgrims tread the pathway with Christ, yet their journey is also held and sustained by the feminine, by Mary his mother, Mystic Rose of the petaled center and window above. In this crucible, where masculine and feminine are in balance and where love moves, transformation and healing can take place.

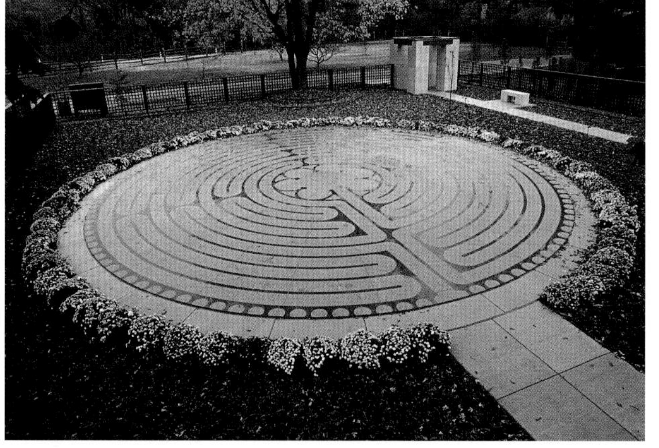

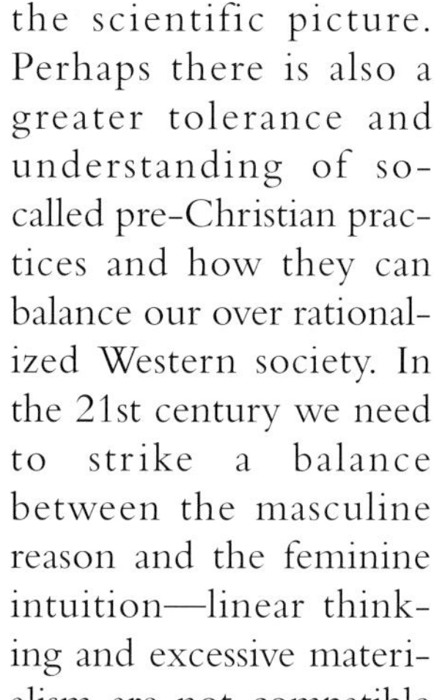

The labyrinth peaked in popularity around the late 15th century, after which it gradually fell out of favor. Indeed, a number of church labyrinths were destroyed in the 18th and 19th centuries. Around this time garden mazes came into vogue, which were used as entertaining mind puzzles and contributed to the demise of the unicursal path. Perhaps too, with the Age of Reason and the rise of linear thinking in philosophy and science, the cyclical and circuitous shape of the labyrinth design seemed out of place.

It was only in the late 19th century that interest in the unicursal labyrinth re-emerged. Its revival might have been aided by modern scientific discoveries, such as electromagnetic waves or coiling strands of DNA, which have put back the curves, twists, and turns in the scientific picture. Perhaps there is also a greater tolerance and understanding of so-called pre-Christian practices and how they can balance our over rationalized Western society. In the 21st century we need to strike a balance between the masculine reason and the feminine intuition—linear thinking and excessive materialism are not compatible with the survival of Earth. The labyrinth balances opposites and brings relief to the deep spiritual drought of our times: its path is curved expressing the feminine, the fixed turning points, where movement almost stops, the masculine. Here we experience the two forces working in harmony, which can be deeply satisfying and healing. Walking its powerful coils also offers us personal space and time to meditate outside our busy schedules, which re-energizes and renews us. Chapters Two to Four will explore how best to access these meditative and healing powers.

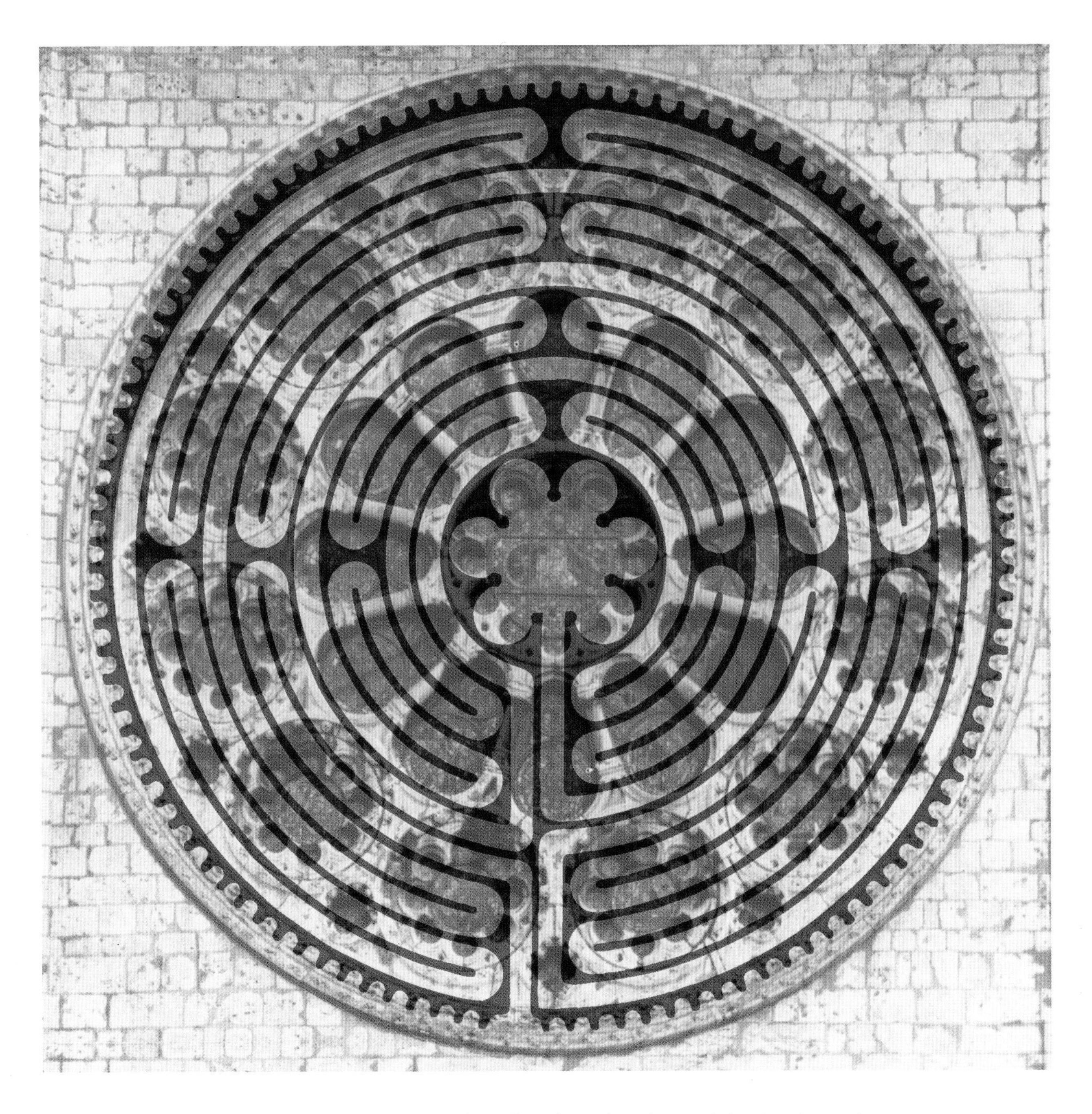

Above: The Chartres labyrinth as if superimposed over the rose window above the west door.

Facing page: New Harmony labyrinth, Indiana. This granite replica of the Chartres design is domed to allow rainwater to run off freely.

2

Preparing the Ground

Your intention to use a labyrinth is the starting point of your journey. Whether the labyrinth you use is merely a small, simple sketch to trace with your finger or a larger, more elaborate design to walk, either alone or as part of a group, certain factors will help to bring your experience to life. If you orient your labyrinth in space, among people and in time, it will become a strong container for your journey. This chapter introduces you to ways in which you can prepare each of these dimensions.

Preparing the space

Of the three dimensions, the most important is your attention to the physical space in which you place or find your labyrinth. Tune in to the present moment with each of your senses—to the sound of the wind in a woodland clearing or to the waves brushing against sand on a beach; to smells of incense in a room or of flowers and grass outside; to colors in the landscape or the quality of light; to the feeling of your heartbeat inside your body or each breath entering your lungs. The combination of your intention and attention means that the labyrinth space will become sacred and powerful, as will your experience in it.

If you are treading an existing indoor or outdoor labyrinth, be it cut in turf or made of stone or brick, all you have to do is attune yourself to its setting in the way described above. If you want to create an indoor or outdoor labyrinth, become attentive to the setting by quietly walking round it. Ask permission of the place you want to use and see if it makes you feel welcome. The answer may be extremely subtle: you might hear the sudden rustling of branches in the breeze or just have a gut feeling that you are in the right place. Respond to your initial reaction, as your instinct will usually sense the quality of the space you have singled out. If the place seems closed to you, there may be something you need to do before entering it. In one location I bathed my hands and feet in a nearby spring before I continued. It is very important that you feel at one with the space you have chosen.

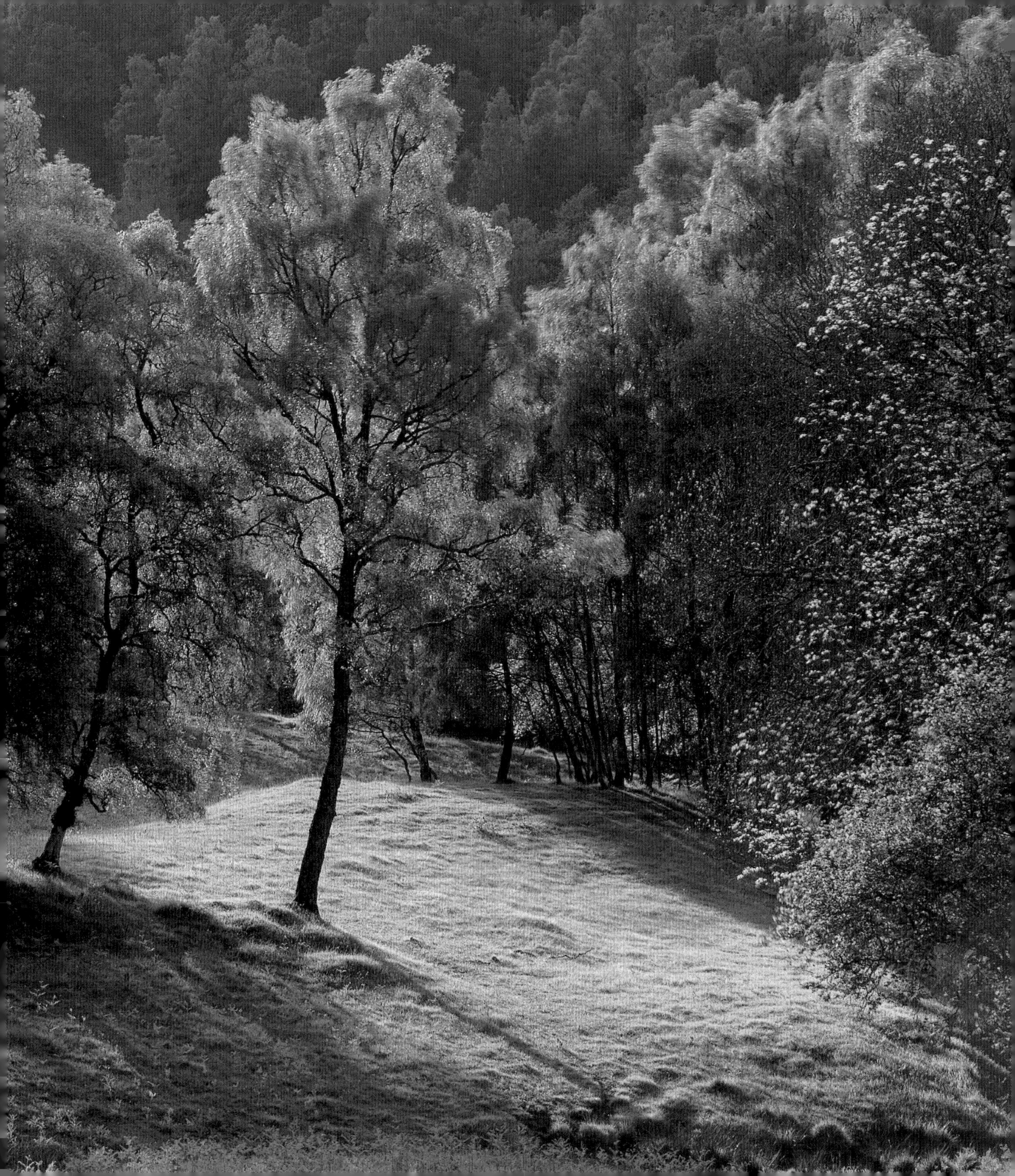

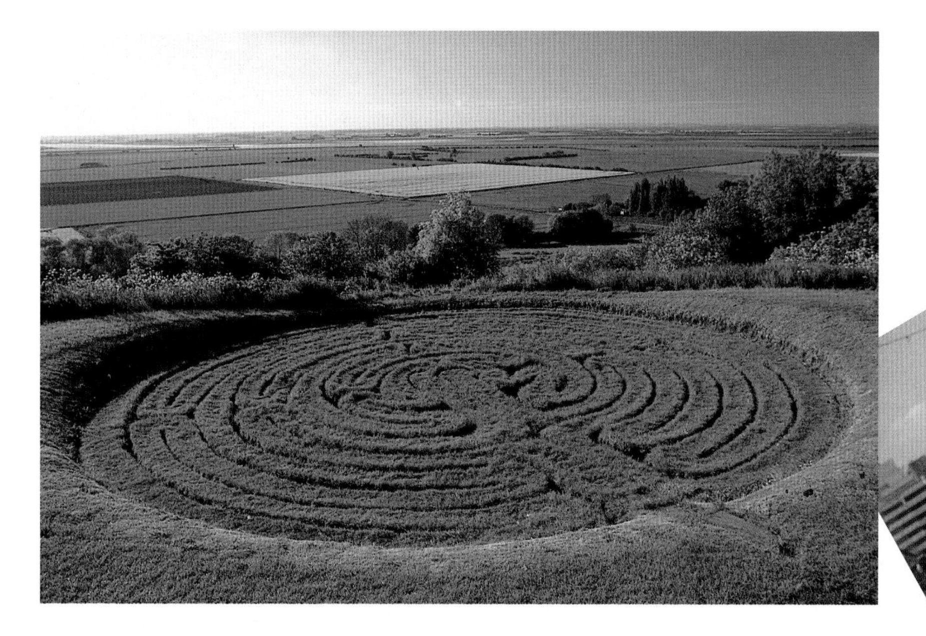

You now need to decide where to lay the entrance pathway to the labyrinth. If you are inside a church or hall and, for instance, want to use the Chartres labyrinth copied on to canvas, you could place this on the east–west axis of the space. You will then face east as you enter the labyrinth, duplicating the orientation at Chartres. Attention to this orientation process will help to draw a spiraling matrix of energy into your space, which can be lost with a canvas copy when the design is away from the strong, protecting stone pillars, soaring roof and jeweled light. Alternatively, you might like to orient your labyrinth using another system you feel comfortable with. In India, for example, cosmic energy, or *prana*, is thought to flow from the northeast toward the southwest, so you could align the entrance/exit pathway with this flow. Try not to get too fixed on any one system: let the labyrinth guide you.

You can also align the entrance of the labyrinth with a key feature of the space you intend to use, so that you look at it as you are about to enter the labyrinth (thereafter you will probably find that your eyes are on your feet). This might be a window with an expansive view of windswept trees in autumn or a particular landmark. You could choose an altar inside a church or create a seasonal table decorated with colors and objects for that time of year, such as pumpkins, apples, and a wooden owl for Halloween, or jugs of milk for Candlemas/Feast of Brigid in February. Palms and purple cloth would mark Lent, and a golden cloth, daffodils, and painted eggs, Easter. Corn dolls, sheaves of ripe wheat, and loaves of plaited bread would honor harvest/autumn. For an individual meditation space at home, where you might trace a labyrinth with your finger, you could place your favorite crystals, important photographs, pictures, or icons together with flowers or candles at the focus-point. The orientation you choose will help create a potent space around the labyrinth.

If you are outside preparing to mow a labyrinth in the grass or chalking one on a playground,

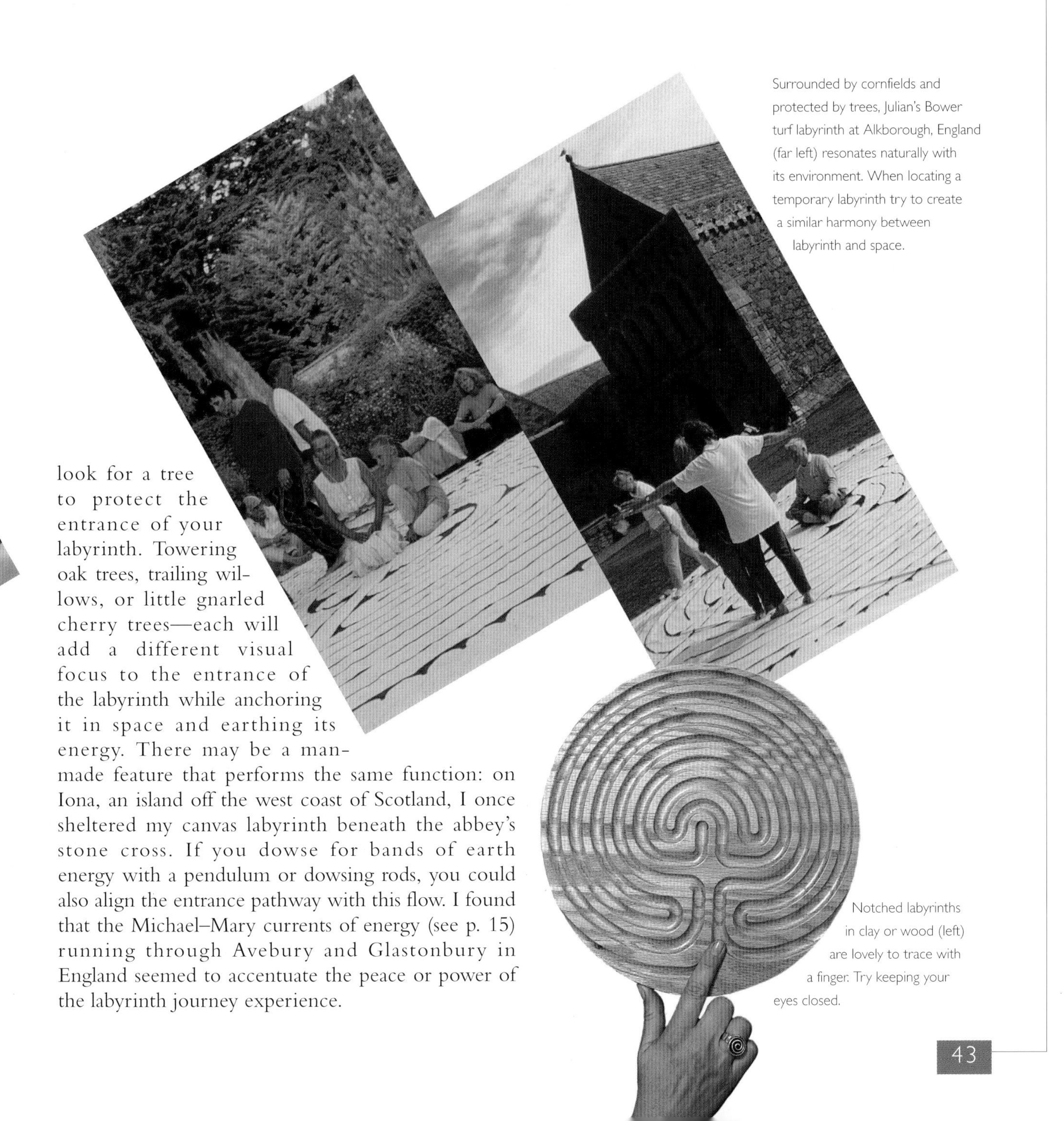

Surrounded by cornfields and protected by trees, Julian's Bower turf labyrinth at Alkborough, England (far left) resonates naturally with its environment. When locating a temporary labyrinth try to create a similar harmony between labyrinth and space.

look for a tree to protect the entrance of your labyrinth. Towering oak trees, trailing willows, or little gnarled cherry trees—each will add a different visual focus to the entrance of the labyrinth while anchoring it in space and earthing its energy. There may be a man-made feature that performs the same function: on Iona, an island off the west coast of Scotland, I once sheltered my canvas labyrinth beneath the abbey's stone cross. If you dowse for bands of earth energy with a pendulum or dowsing rods, you could also align the entrance pathway with this flow. I found that the Michael–Mary currents of energy (see p. 15) running through Avebury and Glastonbury in England seemed to accentuate the peace or power of the labyrinth journey experience.

Notched labyrinths in clay or wood (left) are lovely to trace with a finger. Try keeping your eyes closed.

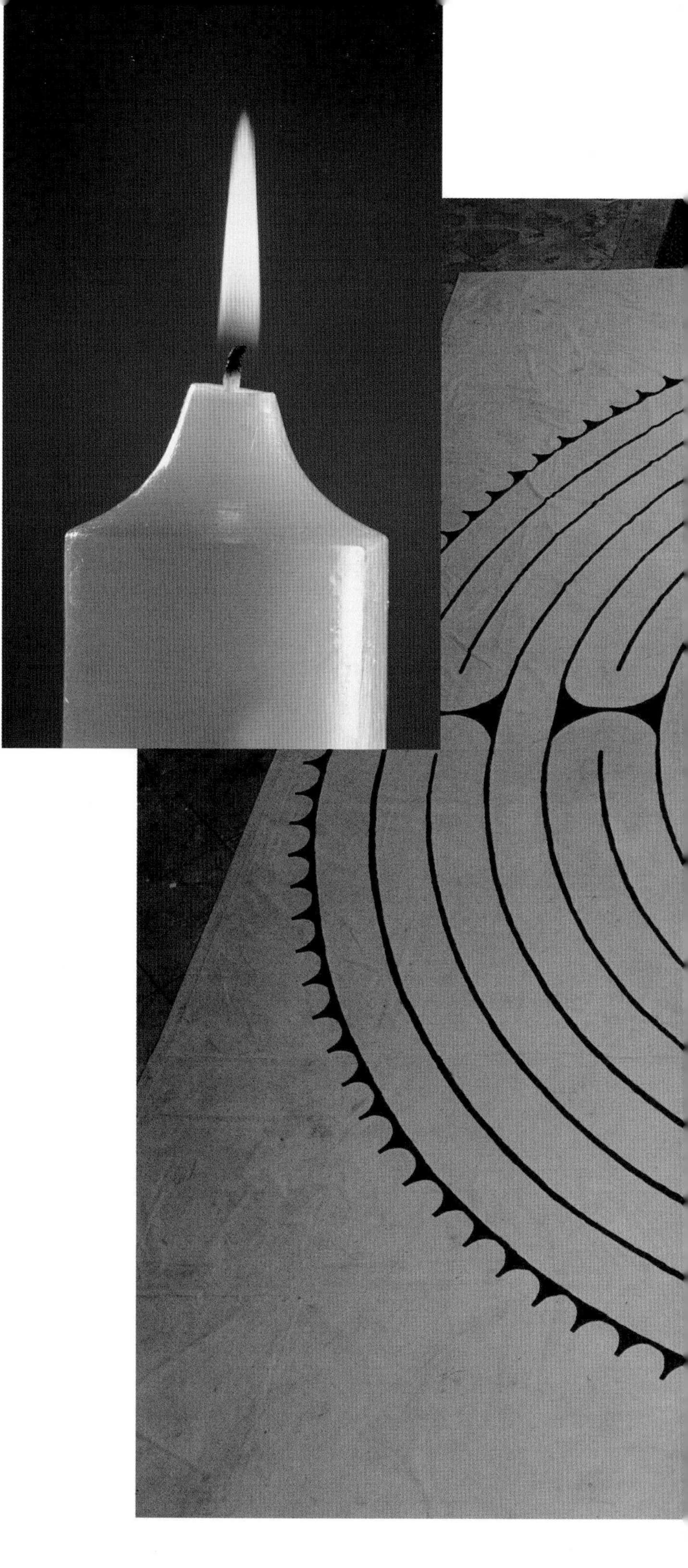

Fire energies

Even when positioned, your labyrinth can still look flat and lifeless. If you light four outdoor flare candles and place one at each corner or on the extended diagonals of a circular-shaped labyrinth, you will find that they pin the canvas down in space and give it invisible, protective walls. Fire brings protection because it creates a boundary: outside the space is ordinary; inside lies the special, sacred space of the labyrinth.

The four sides of the boundary form the shape of a square, which represents the Earth, wholeness, and solidity. You can use this shape to honor the four directions, north, south, east, and west, by moving around the labyrinth and turning to face each one as you light the corresponding candle. You can also call in the four elements—air, fire, water, earth—the four seasons—winter, spring, summer, autumn—and four archangels —Michael, Uriel, Gabriel, and Raphael—and use the four colors—blue, yellow, green, and red.

Naming each side strengthens the sacred space you create. Place four small candles in the center of the labyrinth, bringing them out to each corner before you begin to walk the labyrinth and returning them to the center to be blown out when you have finished. You might like to try a living alternative to candles, with four people holding hands at the center of the labyrinth. They can dedicate the space to the labyrinth pilgrims with a song, dance, prayer, or poem. (I prefer to use the word "pilgrim" rather than "walker," because when the labyrinth is set up ritually, as described in this chapter, the outer journey moves into the dimension of sacred inner and outer space.)

My emphasis on the number four has on occasion shifted to three, the number signifying the soul. At the Chalice Well gardens in Glastonbury (see p. 17) on Millennium Eve, one of the flares broke in two. I

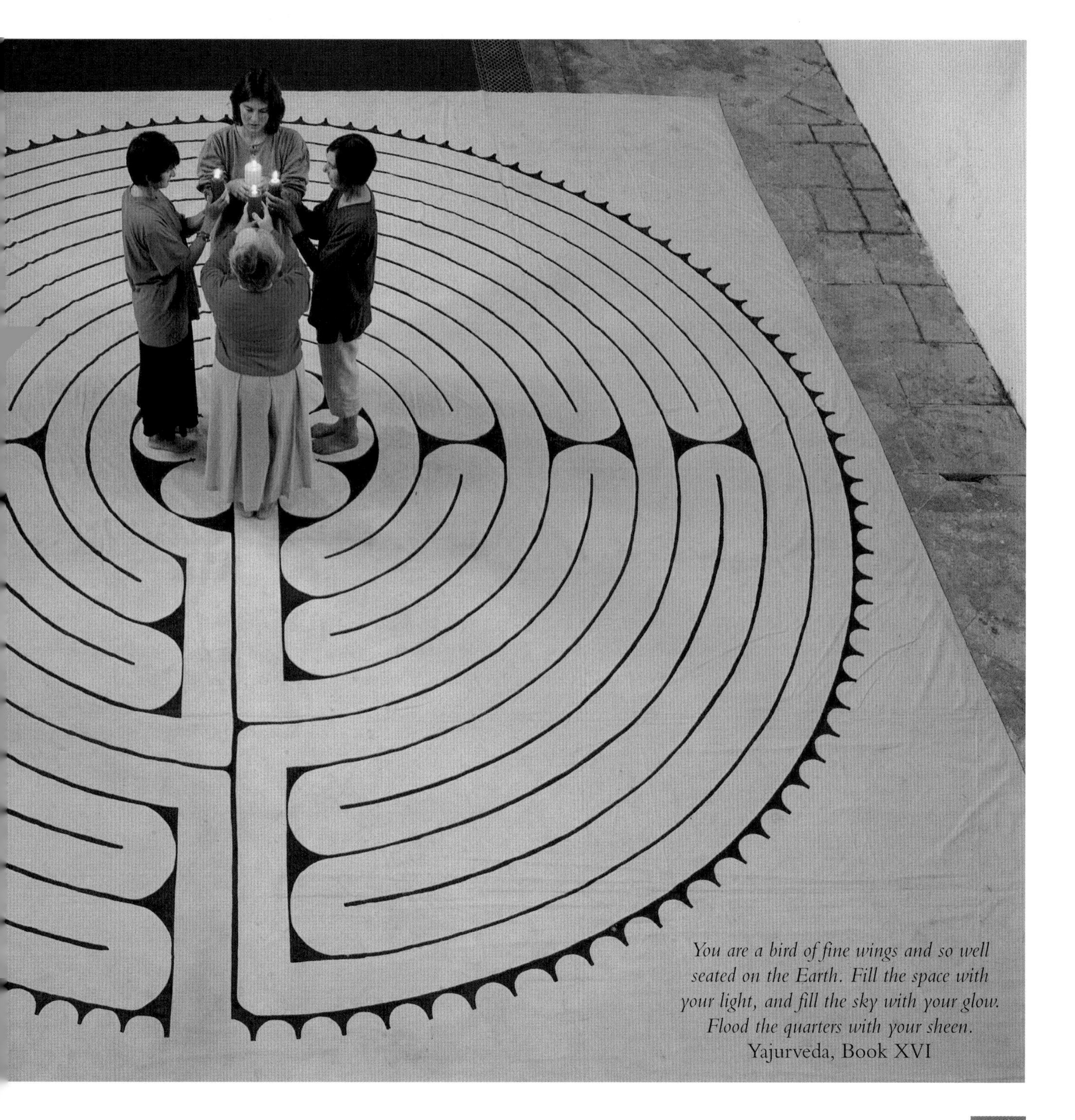

You are a bird of fine wings and so well seated on the Earth. Fill the space with your light, and fill the sky with your glow. Flood the quarters with your sheen.
Yajurveda, Book XVI

decided to plant the two pieces with the last flare and lit them all together just before midnight. The three lit candles brought the feminine archetype of the Triple Goddess, with her three changing faces of Maiden, Mother, and Crone, to that occasion. Her faces link in with the phases of the Moon, full, crescent, and dark. On that night the Goddess showed herself, when quite spontaneously two friends and I joined hands and danced a Greek Circle Dance called *Kore* around the perimeter of the labyrinth. The dance is about Demeter and her daughter Persephone, and the rhythm is in four groups of three beats each. Be attentive to the events surrounding the labyrinth and be flexible in your mind—you may have to change your plans at the last minute.

Fire is also known to cleanse and purify. As the flames on the candles burn, the space between them is purified and made new. Try waving a smudge-stick, a slow-burning compressed bunch of wild sage from the Native American tradition, around the outside of the labyrinth and allow the smoke to drift across it. The smell is pungent and cleansing. You can make your own smudge-sticks with stalks of dried lavender and sage from the garden, bound together with twine.

Human interaction

Once the labyrinth has been anchored in space, you can begin to interact with it. Whether alone or in a group of people, if you dance to music or just move rhythmically around the outer edge of the labyrinth, you will begin to stir its energies and activate both pilgrims and labyrinth for entry. The energy of the space begins to spiral like a whirlpool. I discovered this way of beginning in the abbey grounds at Glastonbury when I was confronted by a large crowd waiting to tread the labyrinth. Knowing my voice could not reach them all, I began walking energetically around

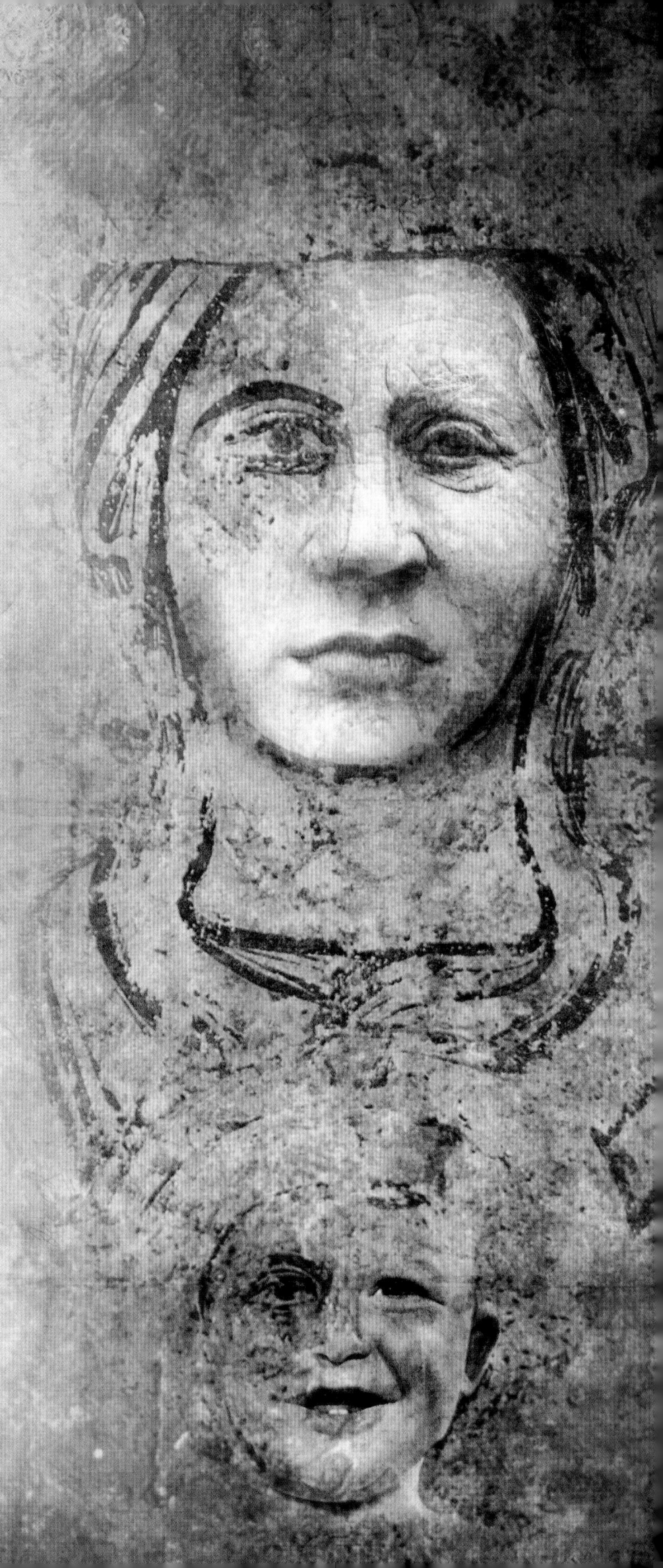

the canvas with my left hand open for people to join on and form a human chain, my right hand beckoning. We danced to the right, the direction of life, until everyone had linked on. Without using my voice or issuing any instructions, a dynamic interaction had begun.

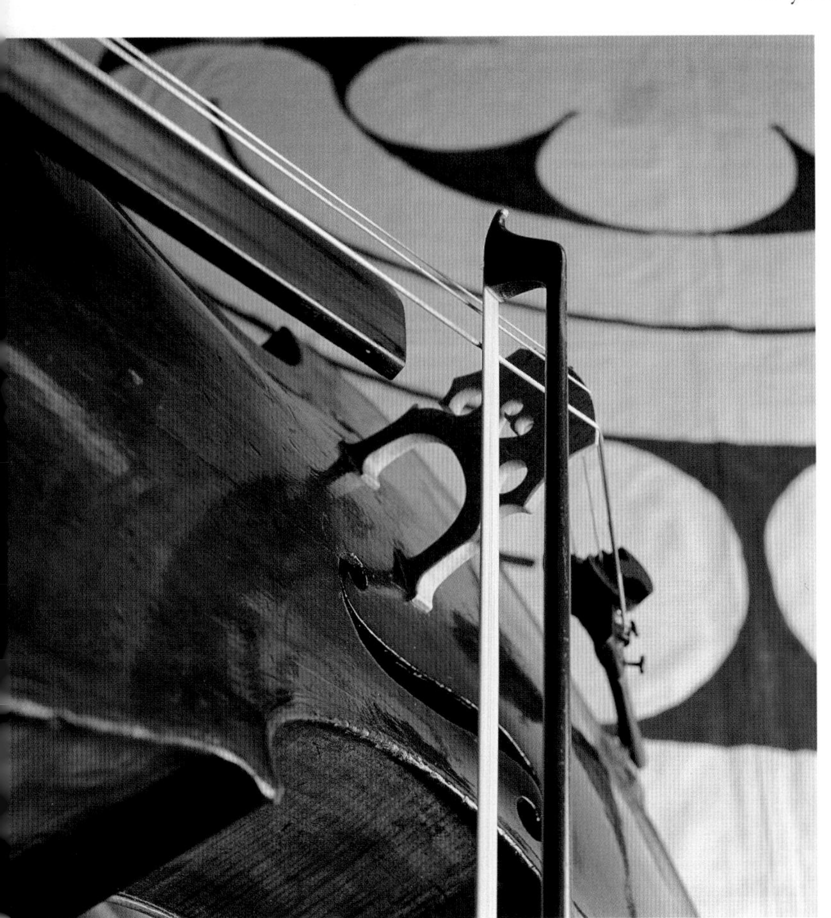

Dances can follow three simple shapes: the circle, the spiral, and the horseshoe (see pp. 48–49). If you are part of a group of pilgrims, the simplest dance is to hold hands in a circle with your right palm up and your left palm down. Walk rhythmically to the right and, at the end of the musical phrase, change direction to the left. Whichever dance you decide on, the most important thing is to enjoy its vitality.

Music on the labyrinth

Music fills the atmosphere and brings harmony to the individual pilgrim or group. When you select your music, you need to choose something that will complement the place and the type of labyrinth you are using. You can dance to it to warm up the space or play it as you journey through the labyrinth. Music with a strong woman's voice, such as Márta Sebestyén from Hungary and Jennifer Berezan (see Resources), works well on the Chartres labyrinth because of its associations with the feminine—the cathedral is dedicated to Mary, Mother of Christ. The Chartres labyrinth has also inspired me to locate medieval songs and dances written in her name. I find that Irish traditional music often suits many Celtic Christian sites, whereas Greek traditional music connects me to the ancient roots of the labyrinth and the myth of Theseus and the Minotaur (see p. 32).

Live music, such as the rich sound of a cello (above), or chanting set up a vibration inside and outside the body.

Triple Goddess (left) with the three faces of Maiden, Mother, and Crone.

Dance energy

Dancing will bring energy into the space. The simplest is the circle (right). Move with your right palms up and left palms down. You can add variations, such as walking into the center for four steps, raising the arms, and walking back out again, dropping the arms. The two dances below are an extension of the circle dance and are especially good for creating a sense of group solidarity.

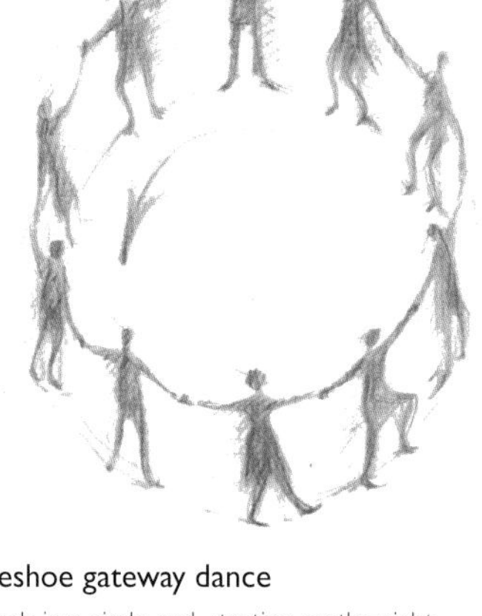

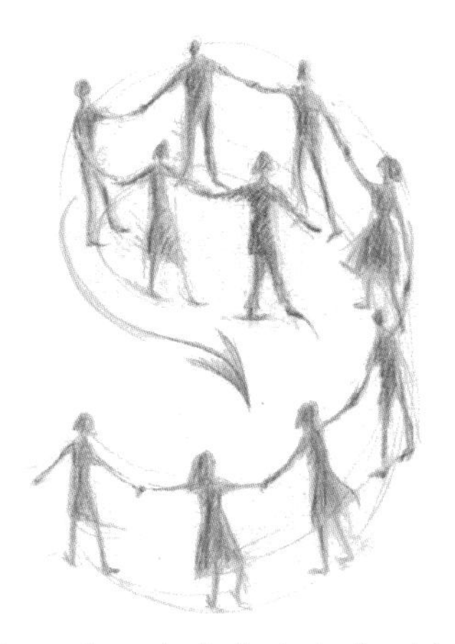

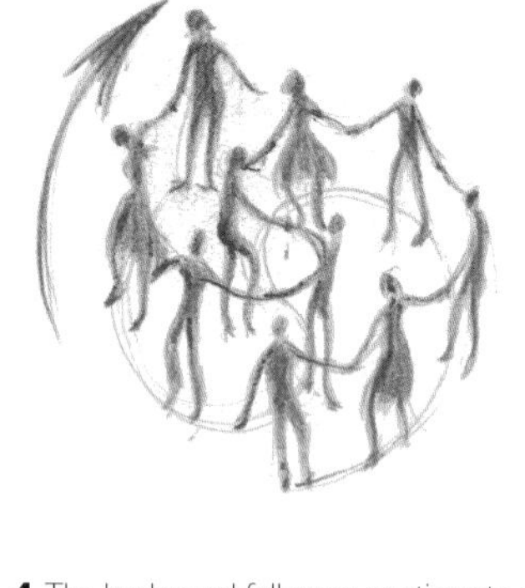

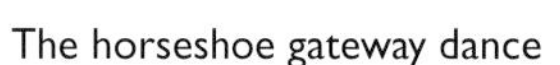

The horseshoe gateway dance

1 Hold hands in a circle and, starting on the right foot, begin to move in a counterclockwise direction.

2 After two or three circuits, the leader (purple) breaks the circle with her/his right hand and turns in on the line of dancers to move in the opposite direction, clockwise, facing the line of dancers. The path will become a horseshoe shape that you follow down on one side and up on the other.

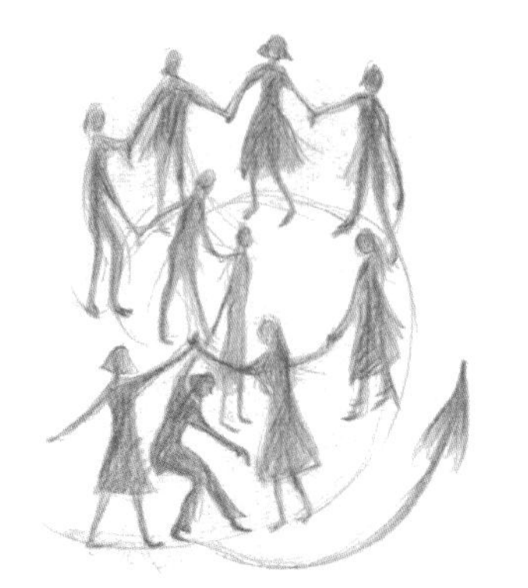

3 When the leader has reached the tail of the circle, the last two people raise their arms to form an arch or gateway for the leader and those following to pass under. Once through the arch, the leader turns to the left.

4 The leader and followers continue to move in a big circle as the loop of people dancing through the arch gets smaller and tighter until, finally, the gate disappears and the dance ends with a complete circle moving around as in step 1.

The beat of the music and the beat of dancing feet echo the vibration pattern of the pathway lines rippling from the center of the labyrinth—a dynamic interaction has begun.

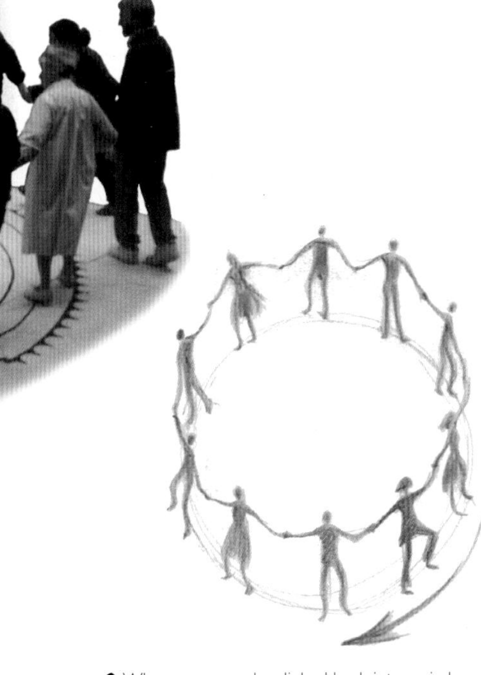

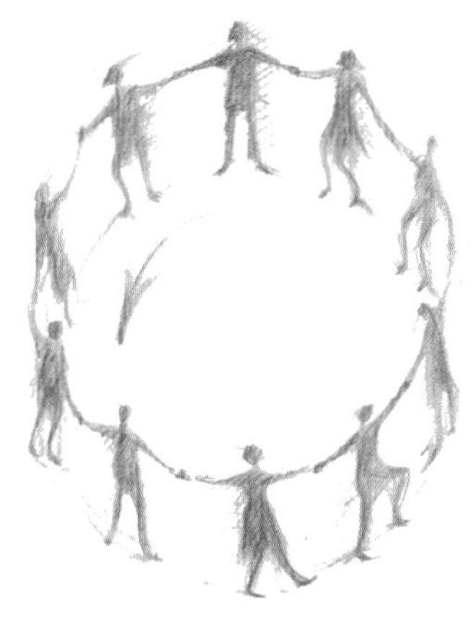

The spiral dance

1 Hold hands in a circle and, starting on the right foot, begin to move in a counterclockwise direction.

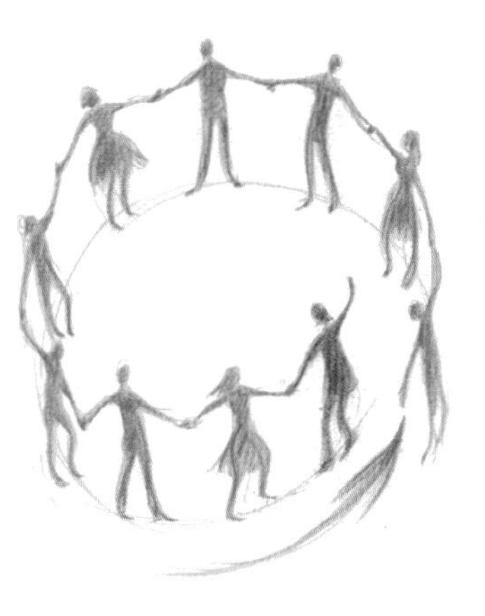

2 The leader (purple) of the dance breaks the circle with her/his right hand and begins to travel on the inner (left) side of the people in front, moving parallel to them, but gradually spiraling inward in tighter and tighter circles.

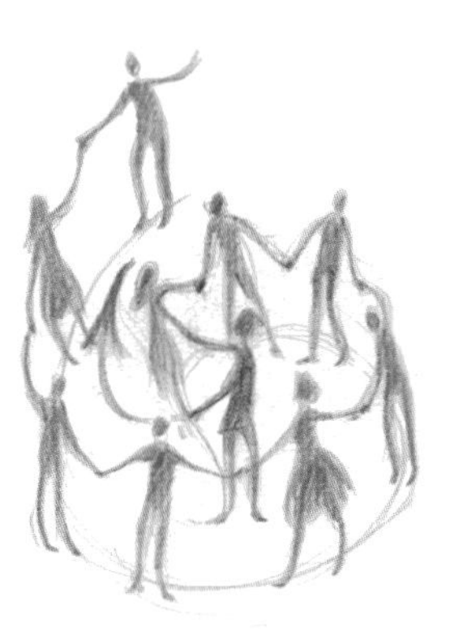

3 The leader continues to draw the other dancers behind him/her until there seems to be no room left at the center. At this point the leader turns sharply on her/his right shoulder.

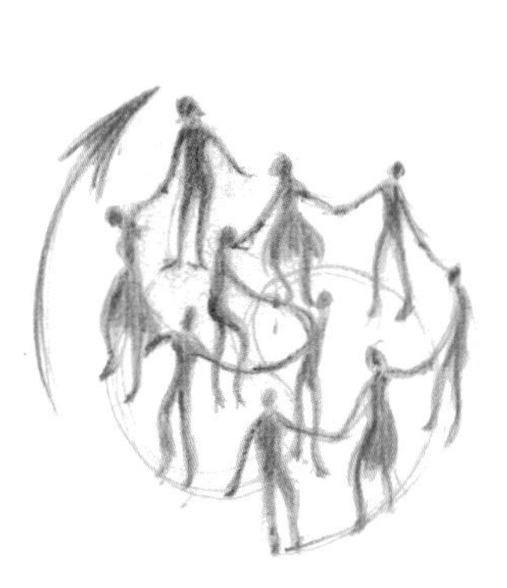

4 The leader then spirals the group out in the opposite direction, passing those still coming into the center.

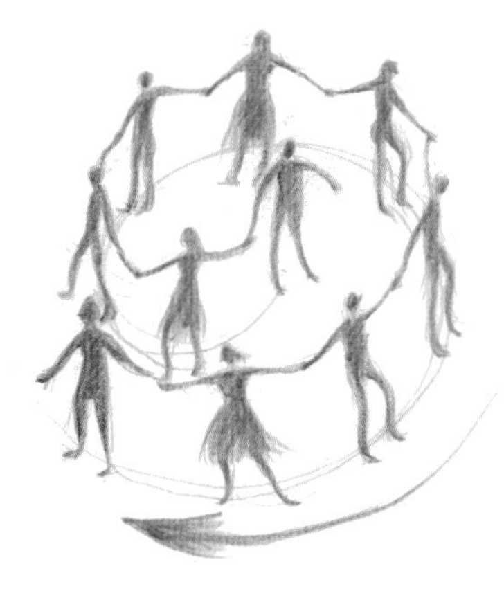

5 All the other dancers follow until the spiral gradually changes back into a circle.

6 When everyone has linked back into a circle they will now be moving in a clockwise direction, the opposite to that at the start of the dance, only this time they will be facing outward.

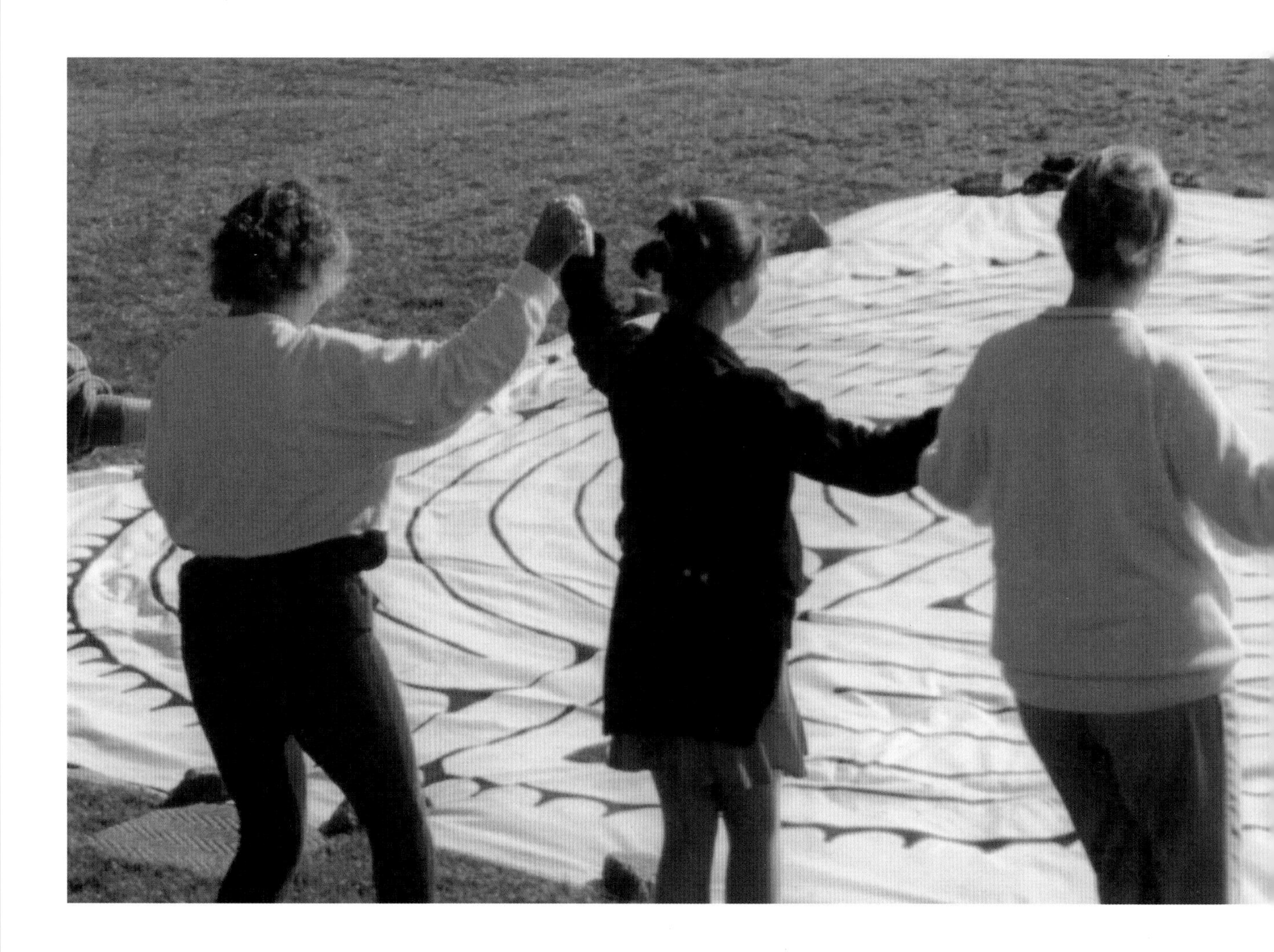

Flame-dancing Spirit, come
Sweep us off our feet and
Dance with us through our days.
Surprise us with your rhythms;
Dare us to try new steps, explore
New patterns and new partnerships;

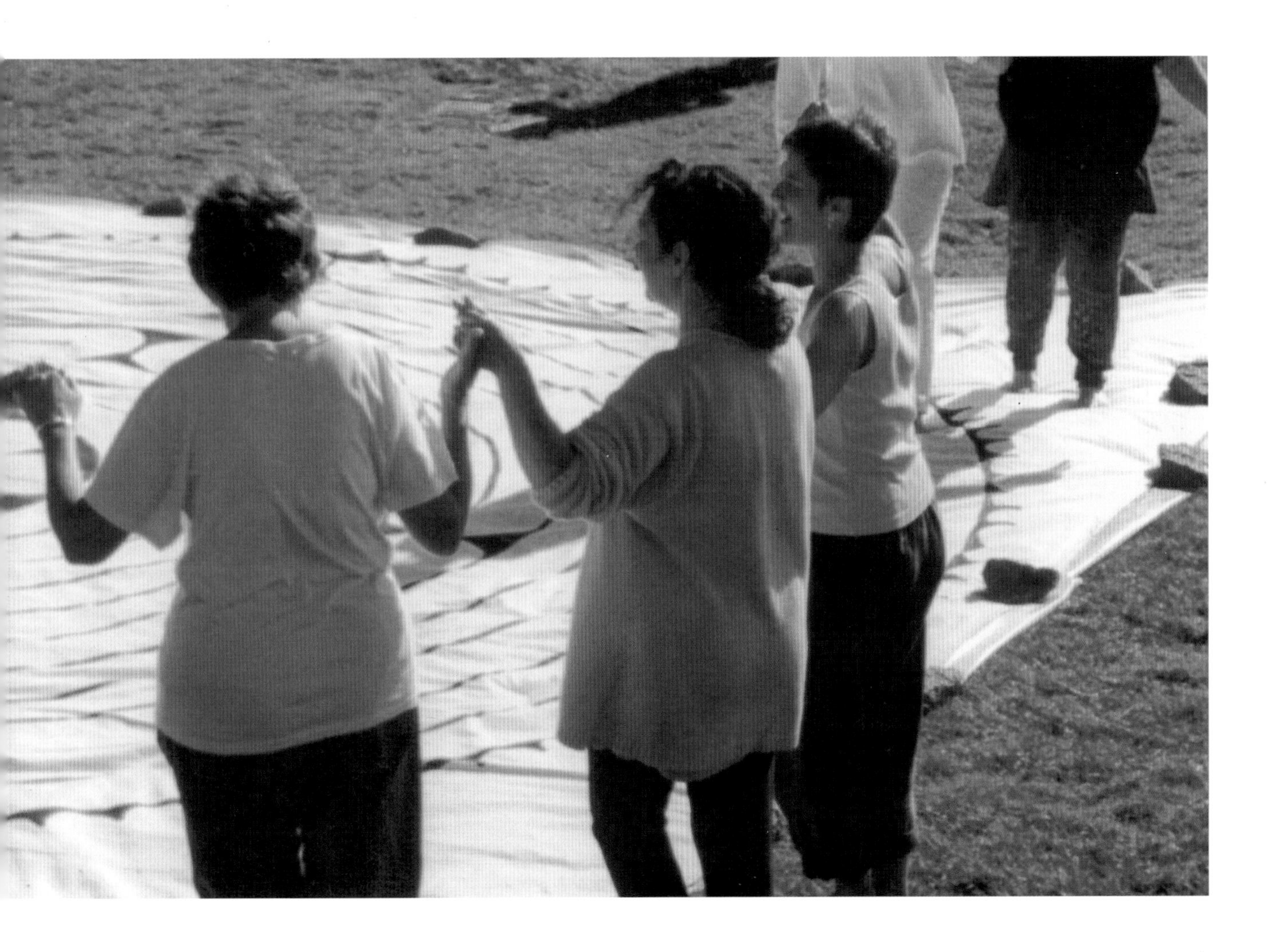

Release us from old routines
To swing in abandoned joy
And fearful adventure.
And in the intervals,
Rest us
In your still center. Ann Lewin

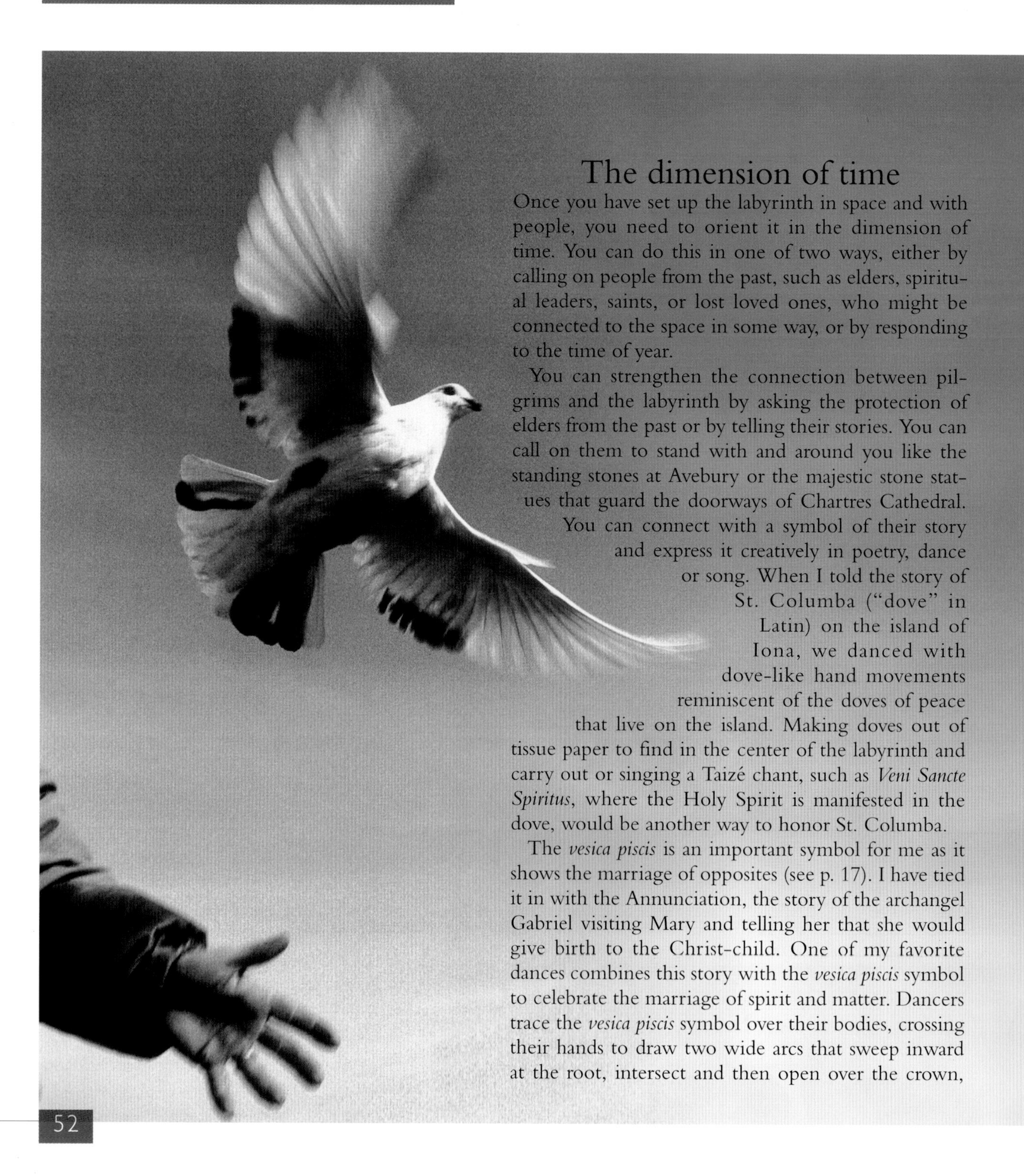

The dimension of time

Once you have set up the labyrinth in space and with people, you need to orient it in the dimension of time. You can do this in one of two ways, either by calling on people from the past, such as elders, spiritual leaders, saints, or lost loved ones, who might be connected to the space in some way, or by responding to the time of year.

You can strengthen the connection between pilgrims and the labyrinth by asking the protection of elders from the past or by telling their stories. You can call on them to stand with and around you like the standing stones at Avebury or the majestic stone statues that guard the doorways of Chartres Cathedral. You can connect with a symbol of their story and express it creatively in poetry, dance or song. When I told the story of St. Columba ("dove" in Latin) on the island of Iona, we danced with dove-like hand movements reminiscent of the doves of peace that live on the island. Making doves out of tissue paper to find in the center of the labyrinth and carry out or singing a Taizé chant, such as *Veni Sancte Spiritus*, where the Holy Spirit is manifested in the dove, would be another way to honor St. Columba.

The *vesica piscis* is an important symbol for me as it shows the marriage of opposites (see p. 17). I have tied it in with the Annunciation, the story of the archangel Gabriel visiting Mary and telling her that she would give birth to the Christ-child. One of my favorite dances combines this story with the *vesica piscis* symbol to celebrate the marriage of spirit and matter. Dancers trace the *vesica piscis* symbol over their bodies, crossing their hands to draw two wide arcs that sweep inward at the root, intersect and then open over the crown, before falling down in a wide circle of wholeness. The movement is set to an English carol called "The angel Gabriel from heav'n did come," which tells the story as the pilgrims dance. Coloring in or writing on enlarged photocopies of the *vesica piscis* is a good activity after this dance.

Alternatively, you can connect the labyrinth in time by thinking of or naming out loud someone who has died and who was very important to you. Perhaps you have a story about him/her that you can share with your fellow pilgrims. You can ask this person to accompany you on your journey through the labyrinth.

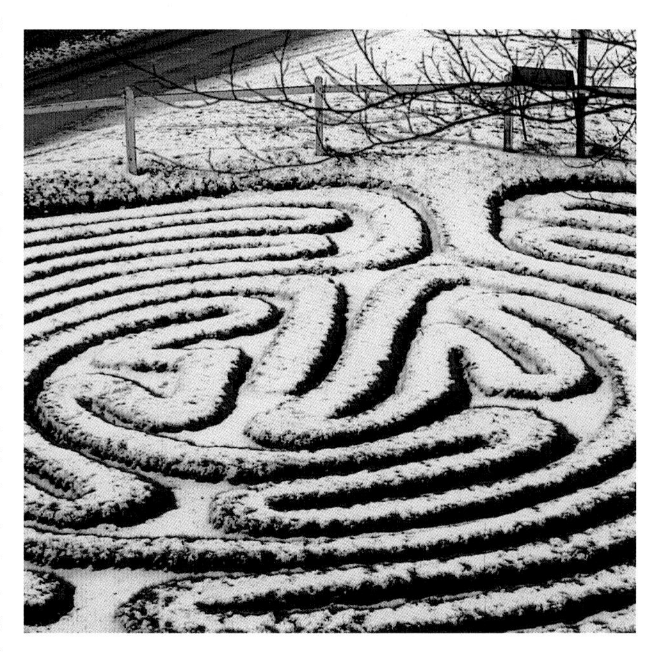

The Wing Maze turf labyrinth in Rutland, England, covered with snow.

If you want to draw out the symbolism of the Theseus and Ariadne story (see p. 32), place a big ball of wool at the entrance of the labyrinth. Before each person begins their journey they can cut off a piece, tie it to their wrist and name a person they want to remember.

Each story you tell and each symbol you explore will reveal another layer of myth and history, as if you and the other labyrinth pilgrims are archeologists excavating for meanings to illuminate the labyrinth. Nothing needs to be rejected, for each layer, be it Christian, Celtic, or Greek, will yield its own treasures.

The labyrinth and cyclic time

You can also tune in to the natural cycle of the year to locate the labyrinth in time. You can do this with a song or a dance that follows the seasons from midwinter to midsummer and back again. You may find that the season of your heart is different from the season or the time of year. It is good to note this and you can take this feeling into the labyrinth with you.

A "Cycle of the Year" dance is a good way to explore this. Play music in the background to suit the mood of the season. Trace a great circle around your torso so that your hands imprint a time map of the sun's path through the year on your body. Different points in this circle represent different times of year. The bottom of the circle where your hands meet is the low point where sap sinks deep into the earth. It is the darkest time of winter, the moment of winter solstice, with the longest night and shortest day. As you raise your arms up to shoulder height you can find a moment of balance. Turn one palm to heaven, the other to earth. This marks spring and the spring equinox, the time of year when the sap quickens and day and night are of equal length. Continue to raise your arms up until they are fully extended above your head. Here you experience the zenith of the seasonal calendar when the sun is at its highest point in the sky. This marks the summer solstice and the longest day and shortest night. As you bring your arms back down again they pass the point of autumn equinox at shoulder height. Day and night are equal once more. And so you return to the lowest point, to the winter solstice, and the cycle starts again.

Thru animate eyes
I divide the seasons of time.

I am aware of what they are.
I am aware of their potential.

With my mouth
I kiss my own chosen creation.
I uniquely, lovingly embrace every image
I have made out of the earth's clay

With a fiery spirit
I transform it into a body
to serve all the world.
Hildegard of Bingen

You can support the movements with your own breath, your lungs empty at the lowest point and full at the highest. Each circle of time that you draw over your body can be subdivided by calling out the names of the Christian or Celtic festivals that take place throughout the year, bringing the two traditions together. In this way, as your arms sweep up in the circle, you explore the layers of time and allow the different festivals to illuminate each other. A rough correspondence can thus be found between the winter solstice and Christmas in December; the feast of Brigid, or Imbolc, and Candlemas in February; the spring equinox and Good Friday in March/April; Beltane, the fire festival, and Easter in late spring; the summer solstice and the Pentecost in June; Lammas, the autumn equinox, and Harvest Festival in late summer; and Samhain (Halloween) and All Saints' Day in October/November. Usually, in a group I name the festivals out loud although the names eventually fade out as you find your particular season in the quiet of your soul, resting in the expression of it through movement.

Now that the labyrinth is strongly oriented in space, among people and in time, you can stand on the threshold of the labyrinth, ready to make your own hero's or heroine's journey to the center.

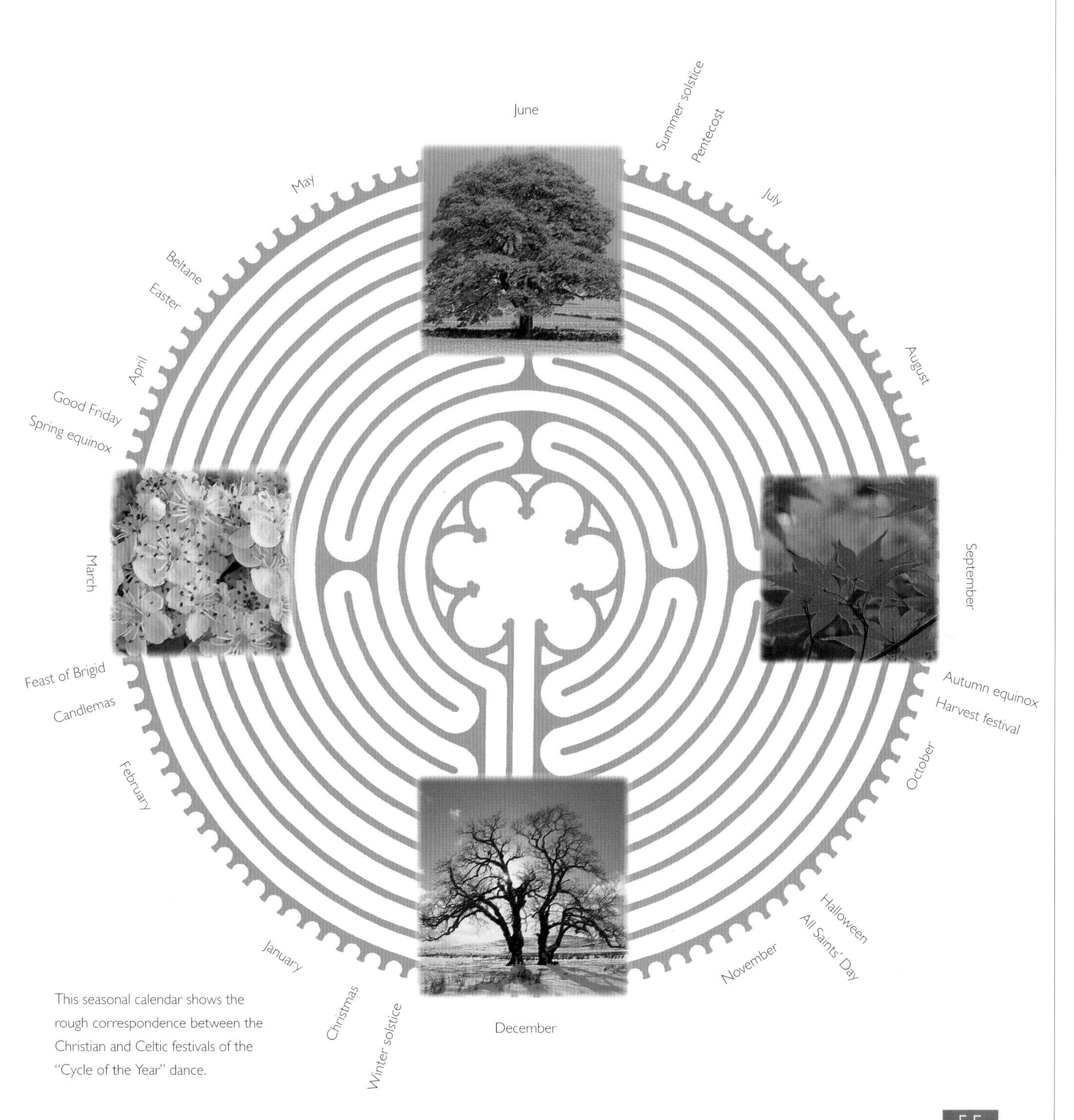

This seasonal calendar shows the rough correspondence between the Christian and Celtic festivals of the "Cycle of the Year" dance.

3

JOURNEY TO THE HEART

At the center, I met myself waiting there for me...
Reflection from a labyrinth pilgrim

Now you have located the labyrinth strongly in space, with people and in time, moving around its circumference to make the energy spiral up into the sky and down into the earth, you are ready to make your journey. This chapter offers suggestions as to how you can follow the path of the labyrinth. You will find that different rituals will appeal each time you tread the labyrinth, for each journey is unique and will influence you in different ways. Open your heart and mind on the labyrinth and let the energy of its coiling pathways flow through your body.

As I mentioned in Chapter Two, if you do not have a large-scale labyrinth available for use you can slowly trace the journey on a picture of a labyrinth with a finger of your nonwriting hand. You can either draw a classical labyrinth (see pp. 88–89) or use the copy of the Chartres design on p. 96.

The four movements

The labyrinth journey can be divided into four movements: "on the threshold," "journeying in," "the resting place," and "journeying out." Each movement adds a new element to your experience: waiting and gathering yourself at the threshold gives way to movement and to realizing who you are at that moment; your journey in opens your mind and lets thoughts and emotions flow freely; your arrival at the center allows you to rest and opens up the possibility of a new awareness being born; your journey out allows you to return with this awareness. You may find these four stages helpful to interpret your experience; alternatively, you can find other words to assist you.

The majority of this chapter explores individual journeys on the labyrinth, when you are not necessarily alone on the labyrinth, but follow the path at your own pace. Group journeys are a very different and fun experience, so the final pages of this chapter show you how to dance in a long chain of people to the center.

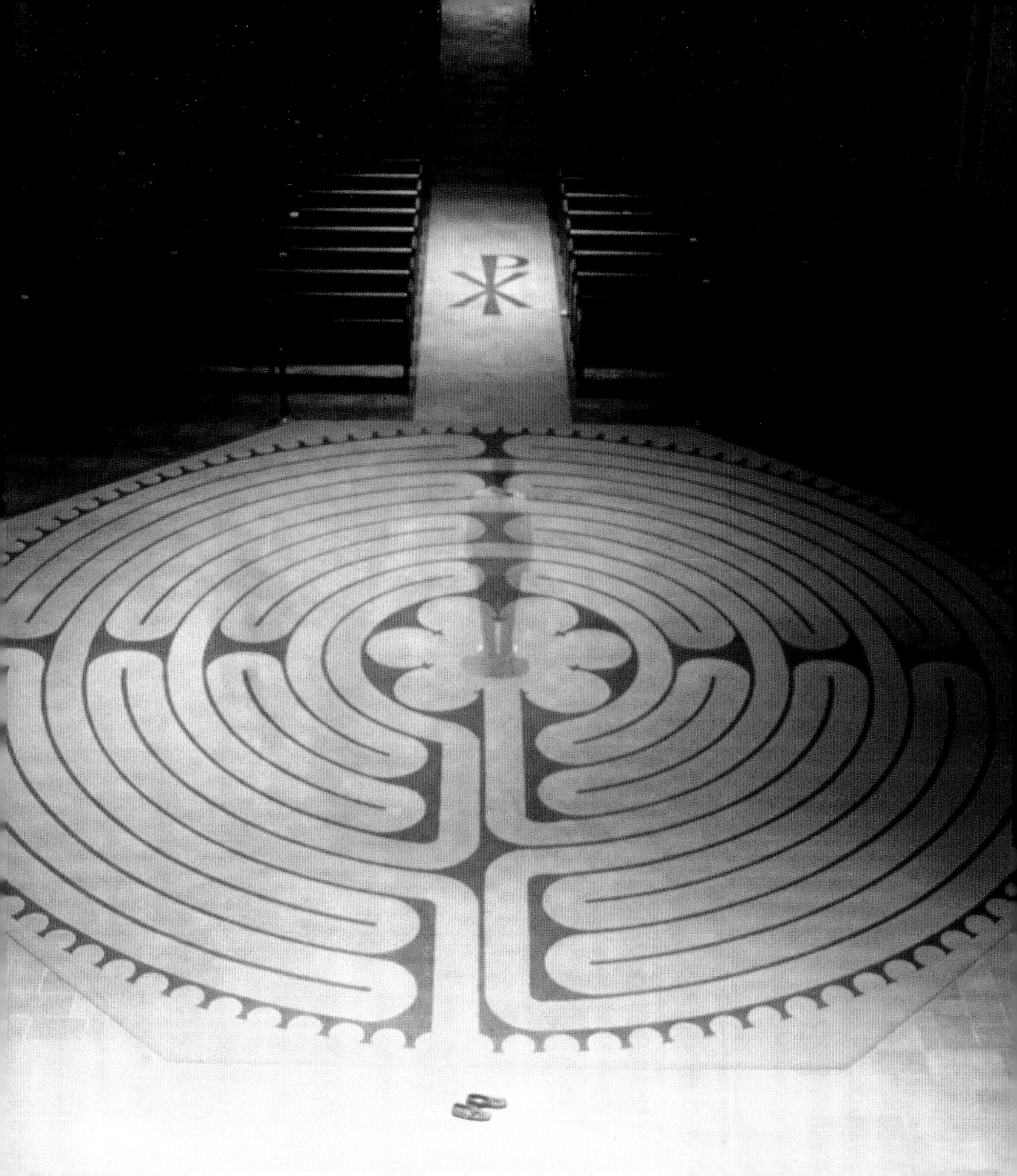

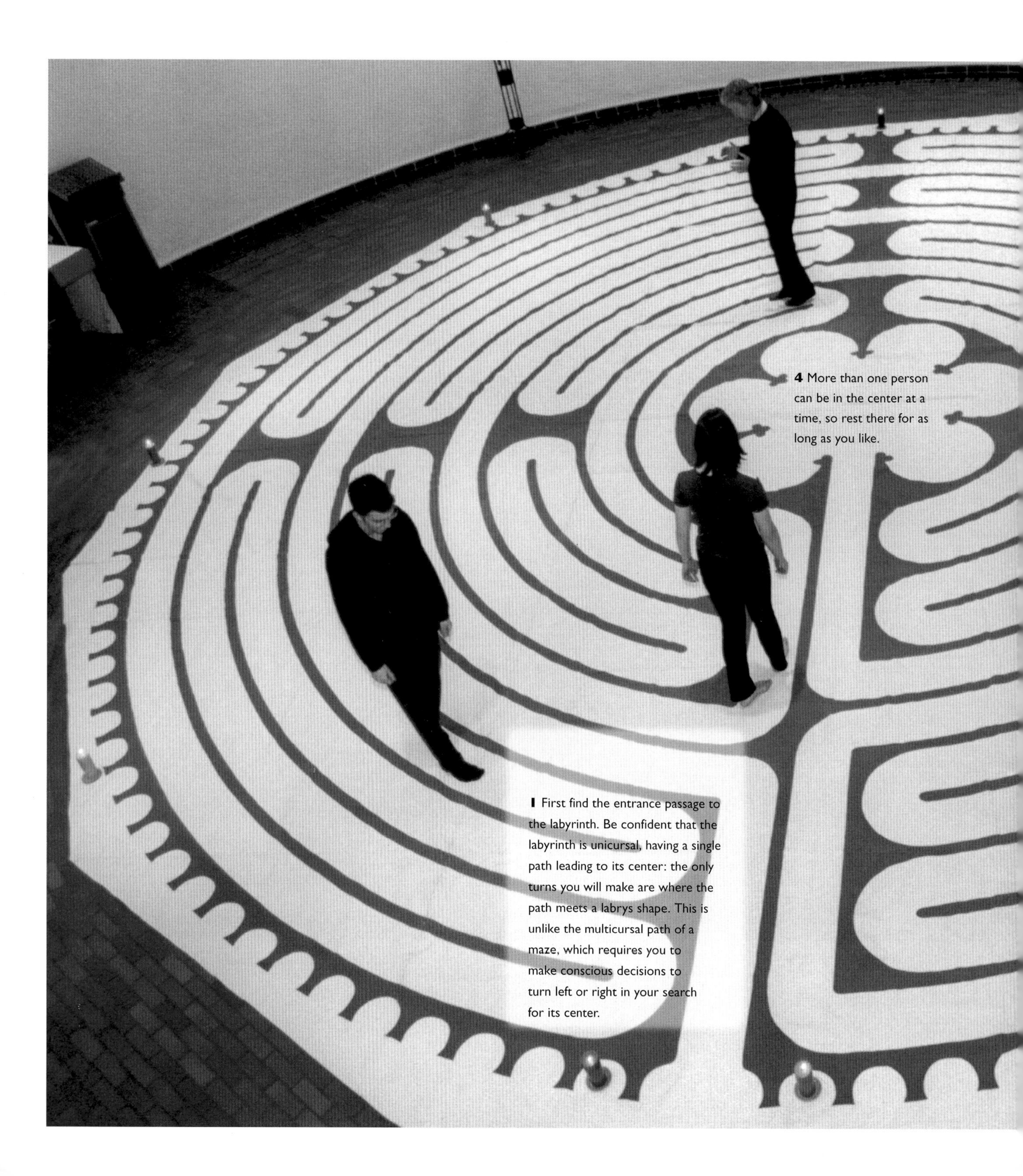

4 More than one person can be in the center at a time, so rest there for as long as you like.

1 First find the entrance passage to the labyrinth. Be confident that the labyrinth is unicursal, having a single path leading to its center: the only turns you will make are where the path meets a labrys shape. This is unlike the multicursal path of a maze, which requires you to make conscious decisions to turn left or right in your search for its center.

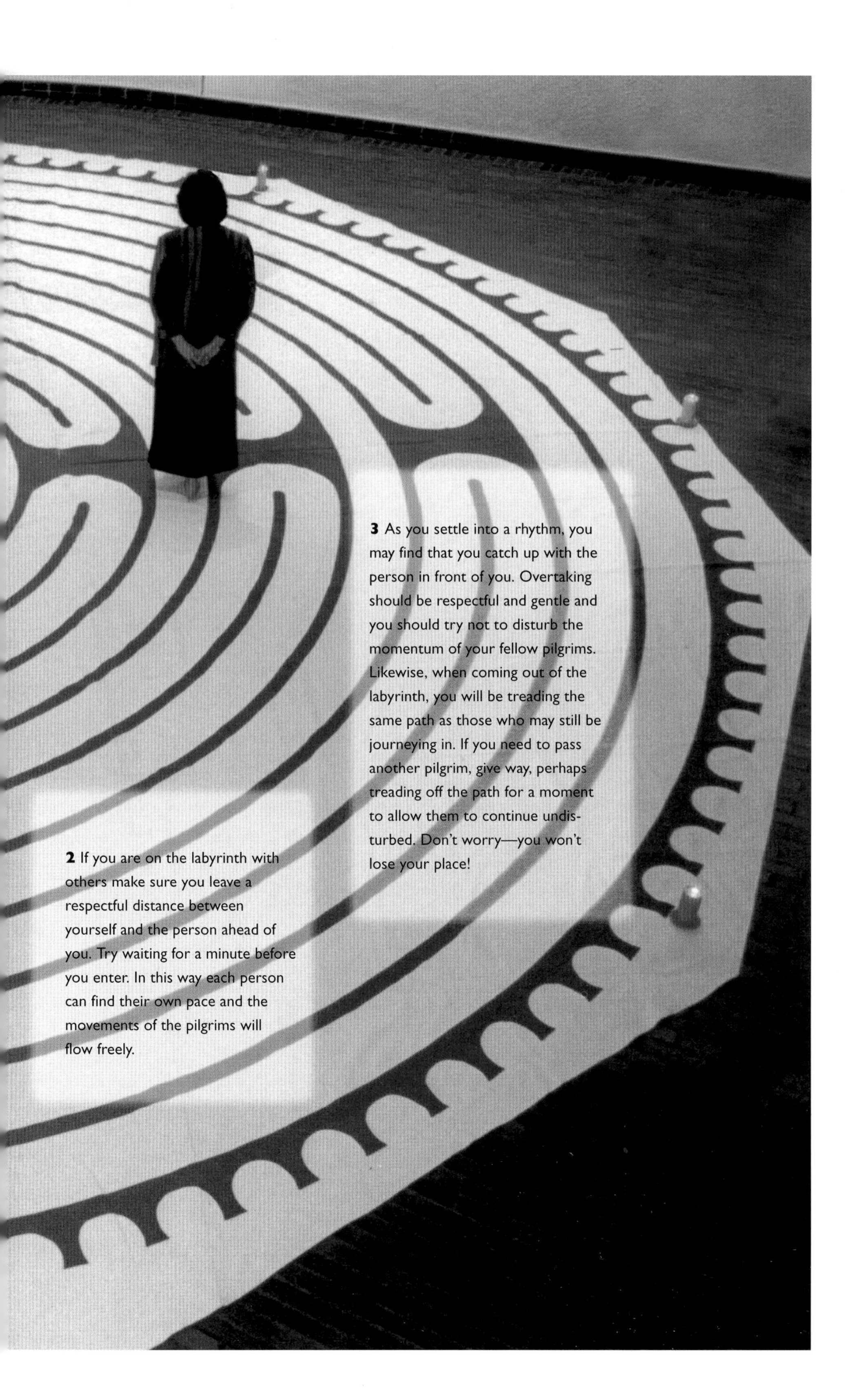

3 As you settle into a rhythm, you may find that you catch up with the person in front of you. Overtaking should be respectful and gentle and you should try not to disturb the momentum of your fellow pilgrims. Likewise, when coming out of the labyrinth, you will be treading the same path as those who may still be journeying in. If you need to pass another pilgrim, give way, perhaps treading off the path for a moment to allow them to continue undisturbed. Don't worry—you won't lose your place!

2 If you are on the labyrinth with others make sure you leave a respectful distance between yourself and the person ahead of you. Try waiting for a minute before you enter. In this way each person can find their own pace and the movements of the pilgrims will flow freely.

Organizing a group

If there are a number of you wishing to walk the labyrinth, you should think about how many of you will fit comfortably on its path without encroaching on each other's space. The labyrinth I use on canvas is 21.4 ft. (6.5 m) wide, with 9 inch (23 cm) pathways. For a labyrinth of this size, you will be limited to about 20 people treading it at any one time; more, and there will be a traffic jam effect resulting in frustration and chaos. Instead, you should provide enough structure to allow the pilgrims and labyrinth to interact freely.

With a group of about 40 people, I would ask half to choose one of the four corners of the canvas to sit on, and then give their full attention to those walking the labyrinth as they wait their turn. They perform the valuable task of holding those journeying in their gaze; in their stillness they are the witnesses, an essential part of the movement. They surround the perimeter of the space like a human wall, making it safe for those inside. They can also chant, creating a wall of sound to hold the pilgrims. If a pilgrim needs human contact after their journey, those outside the labyrinth can receive them in silence or with words.

Labyrinth project at the University of Dundee, Scotland. See Resources (pp. 106–109) for details.

On the threshold

Most people take their shoes off before entering the labyrinth. This is a good act of divesting and helps you to connect strongly with the earth and the energies of the labyrinth. Once, at the Chalice Well gardens in Glastonbury, the whole group linked up in a chain and danced barefoot through the shallow pool at the bottom of the water cascade. The shock of the cold water on our feet was invigorating and we felt cleansed as we entered the labyrinth. If there is no spring or pool nearby, use a small bowl of water placed at the entrance of the labyrinth to sprinkle over your head or hands. In the same way, before you trace a small paper labyrinth with your finger, pour cold water from a bowl over your wrists and hands as a cleansing action.

Water flows over these hands.
May I use them skilfully
to preserve our precious planet.
Thich Nhat Hanh

My first ever step into the labyrinth was an emotional moment, and it took me a few seconds to make the next.
Reflection from a labyrinth pilgrim

Pause

Before you begin your labyrinth journey, pause for a moment at the entrance to center yourself. You may want to bend down toward the earth and touch an object that reminds you of the elements and calls you to yourself. Try ringing a small bell or wafting a burning smudge-stick of wild sage around your body (you may prefer it if someone does this for you). Or place ice cubes containing frozen flower buds in a bowl as a symbol for the frozen to be melted. Blowing bubbles with soapy water will bring in air and lightness. Let yourself be filled and emptied by your breath.

As preparation for your journey on the labyrinth, you can refresh your whole body by quietly energizing and opening your chakra system by visualization. The chakras are an ancient Indian system describing energy centers of light and color, like moving wheels, interpenetrating the body at seven key points. These are the sexual root of the torso (corresponding color: red), the sacral area just below the navel (orange), the solar plexus (yellow), the heart (green and pink), the throat (blue), the brow (indigo) and the crown of the head (violet). With each breath visualize translucent color suffusing each chakra, starting at the root, and each chakra opening like the petals of a flower.

As you enter, you might need to find a word, question, prayer, or mantra as a focus for your journey. There might be an angel or guide to call in or you may just wish to clear your mind and be open. The anticipation you feel as you stand at the entrance of the labyrinth might be like that of a diver on the edge of a diving board, looking down into the water below before taking the plunge.

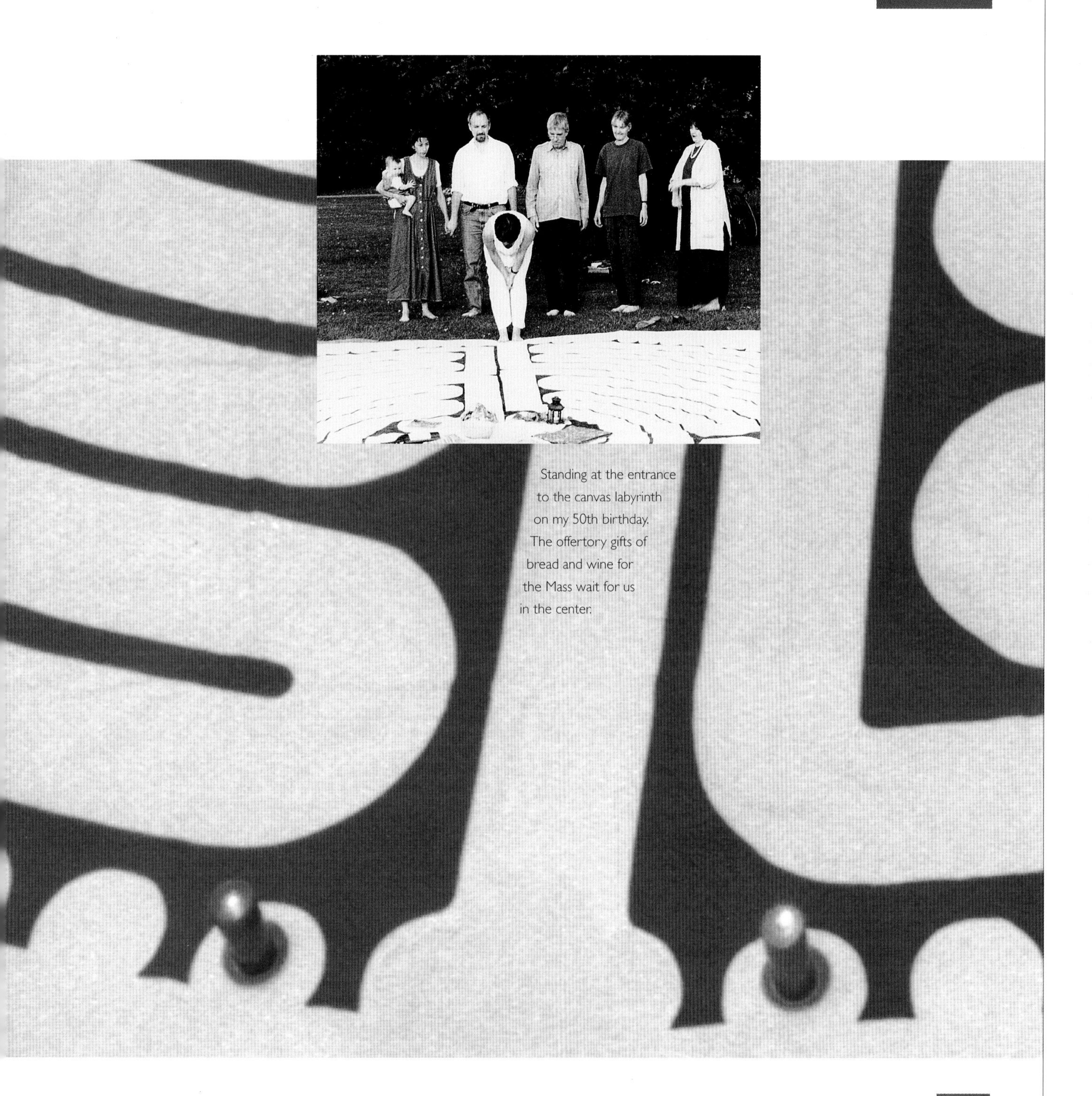

Standing at the entrance to the canvas labyrinth on my 50th birthday. The offertory gifts of bread and wine for the Mass wait for us in the center.

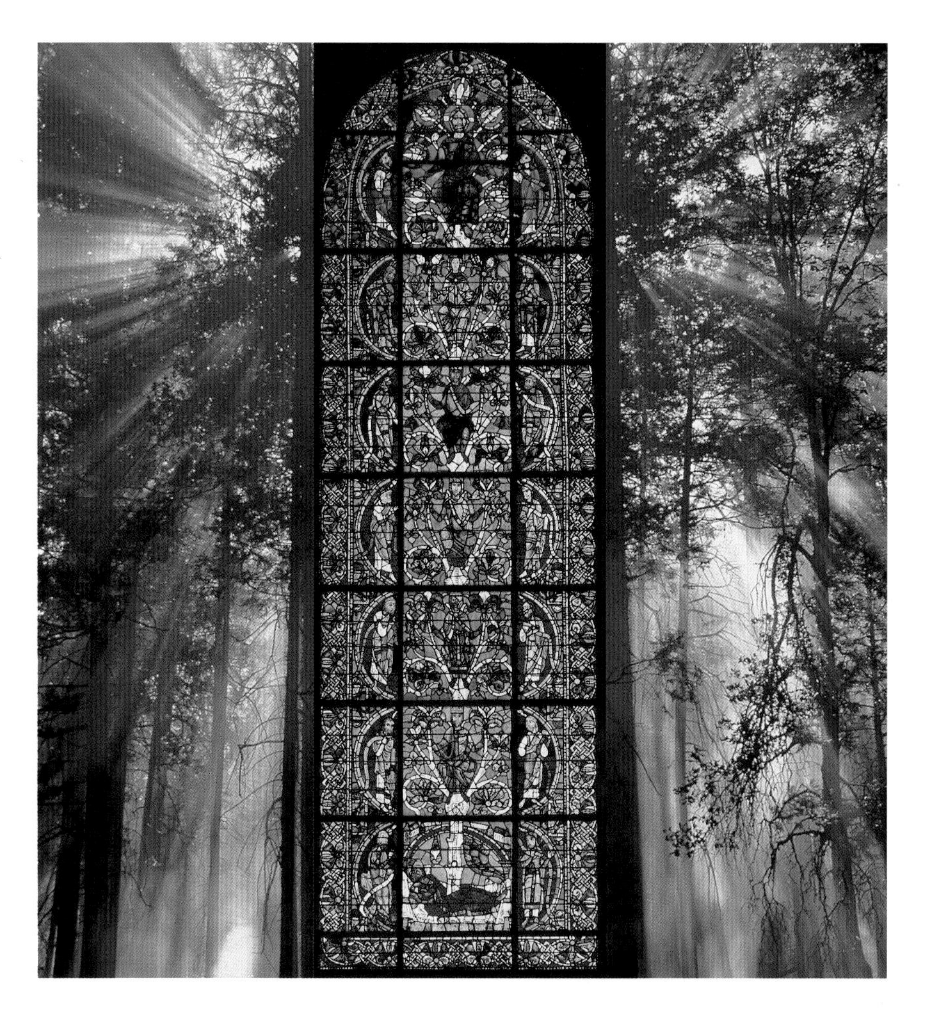

Journeying in

If you have chosen to walk or trace the Chartres labyrinth, you will see as you enter that the path lies straight ahead. It then curves to the left at 90 degrees, sweeping up and then back to the straight path. The shape trodden looks like the trunk of a tree, its branch sweeping up to the heavens. You are climbing the tree, just like the tree seen from the labyrinth if you were in Chartres Cathedral: if you were to look up at the right-hand stained-glass window of the triptych over the west door, you would see the Tree of Jesse. In the Old Testament Jesse is the root, the first in the line of Kings, King David among them, and ancestor of Jesus. The Kings sit on each axil of the tree, resting their feet on the branches that curl up and out on either side of them.

Even if you are not in Chartres Cathedral, this image can be very helpful for your journey on the labyrinth: you are climbing the tree of your own life, stretching back to your ancestors and forward to those yet to be born, and touching the lives of saints and holy people through the ages. You journey alone on the labyrinth, but you are still in the company of figures from your past and present who have touched your life. This is mirrored when there are others with you on the labyrinth: sometimes they are alongside you as if you were in a crowd, often coming straight at you but turning away just before you meet; and at other times you are quite alone. How you perceive the other pilgrims in your heightened state of awareness has a huge impact on your journey and can be a revelation. You may find emotions rising to the surface, such as anxiety ("Will I find my way?") or impatience ("Why is the person in front of me moving so slowly?") or anger ("Why do I always give way to other people on the path?"). Thus the labyrinth acts like a mirror and teacher, telling you something direct about yourself. Try not to suppress feelings that arise as you walk; instead, embrace them. You will have the opportunity to let them go as you make a turn.

If you are treading a classical labyrinth you will enter the middle pathway and explore the outer circumference of the labyrinth in three swings; you will then near the center and eventually enter it after two small swings. In the Chartres labyrinth, after you have climbed the tree, the path takes you close to the center, doubling back and forth around it; you will then gradually move out to the circumference through the four quadrants before sweeping in to the rose-petaled center of the labyrinth.

You will find that following the path of any labyrinth requires just enough concentration to keep the mind busy, particularly the Chartres labyrinth, as the turns are not regular and you have to focus on the path ahead. This gives your being a chance to shed layers of distraction and worry, and the mind an opportunity to stop its chatter. The body's movement is also disorientating as you are absorbed in the movement of your feet and not looking out into space as usual. You will find that your perception sharpens.

As I walked to the center thoughts flowed through my mind, and with each turn another surfaced until layer upon layer of questions, hopes, desires, and tentative solutions filled me, overflowing in the center.

At one point [on the labyrinth] I was deeply moved, as I encountered some darkness inside me; the darkness I didn't really want to see. Then I kept going onward to the light...

The turns

It is easy to lose yourself in the turns of any labyrinth. In the Chartres labyrinth you make twenty-eight 180 degree turns, 13 turning on the left shoulder, and 15 on the right. After the first four turns you make alternate right and left turns in clusters of four left–right turns, then four right–left. This is followed by a long section of ten left–right turns, ending with four right–left and four left–right turns. In the classical seven-path labyrinth you make eight turns, half of these on your right shoulder, the other half on your left. These changes of direction may have a strong effect on the electromagnetic field of the body.

If you look at the shape on the pathway of the Chartres labyrinth that makes the path double back on itself in a fat rounded coil, you will see that it resembles the blade of the labrys, or double-headed axe. This was a symbol of the Minoan civilization, and was thought to represent the bull, which was central to their worship.

Although many historians link the worship of the bull with the Cult of the Dead, some feminists link it with reproduction and fertility, as the shape resembles the womb, ovaries and fallopian tubes. If the Minoans did indeed adopt the axe from the Amazon women, then this theory is not unreasonable. Whichever theory we accept, both tie in with the labyrinth's association with fertility, life, and death (see Chapter One). This is a fitting symbol to find on the labyrinth: not only does it connect the labyrinth with its Ancient Greek roots, the myth of Theseus and the Minotaur, and the themes of birth and death, but it also underlines the effect of cutting and changing that the labyrinth turns have on its pilgrims. Each time the under-edge of the cutting labrys blade slices through the path, you are halted in the direction you are traveling and have to turn around and resume your journey in completely the opposite direction. Use these turns to meditate on as you walk into the center, changing your train of thought or shaving away a layer of worry with each turn.

You bend and sway around the labyrinth and as you move around it, it is impossible to get stuck in one line of thought.

In ordinary life, when you are off the labyrinth, you may find yourself making physical turns with new awareness and enjoyment, such as turning at the end of a lane in the swimming pool or turning a full 180 degrees around the banisters at the top of the stairs. In the same way, enjoying the turns on the labyrinth can help us to accept change in our lives and find new ways to move from one phase to the next. Turns on the labyrinth show us that although change in our lives may feel retrogressive or that we have lost our way, we are actually still moving on toward the central goal. In this way, the labyrinth can be very reassuring, reminding us that life is full of changes that should not be feared but welcomed.

The route reflected many things: sometimes an over-crowded path, sometimes quite alone; the constant reversal of direction, yet inevitably leading to the center; different moods on the way—solemn and light-hearted—and wanting to dance sometimes.

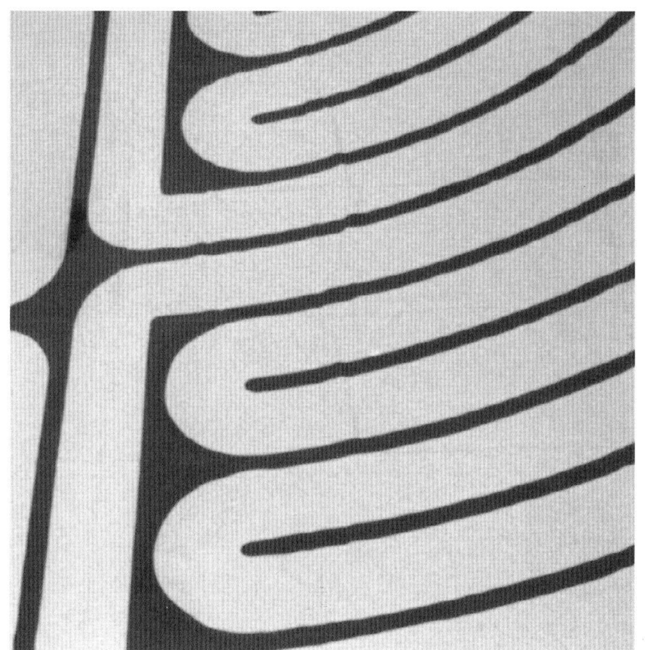

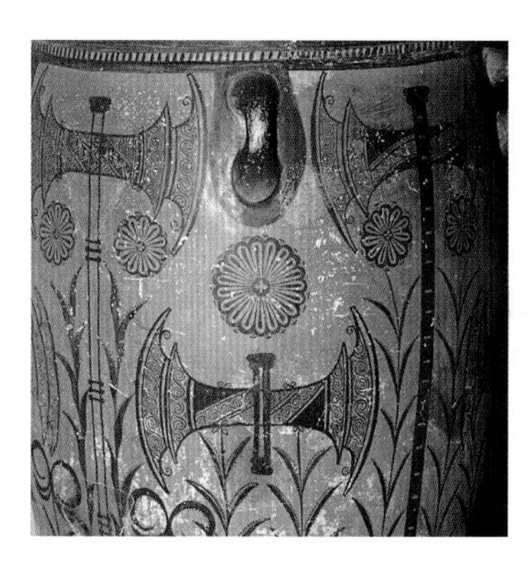

Detail of a labrys design on a pithos from Knossos, Greece, circa 1458–1400 B.C.

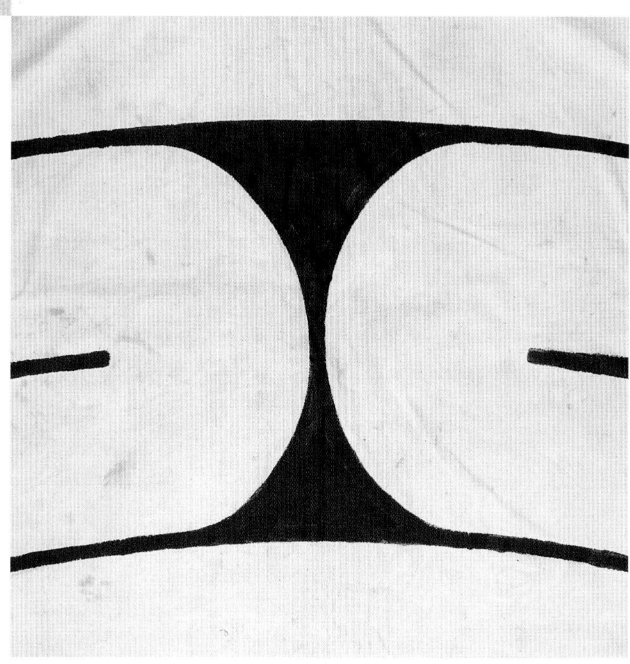

This labyrinth taught me
when you get knocked off your path by others
to stay calm and continue, one step at a time.

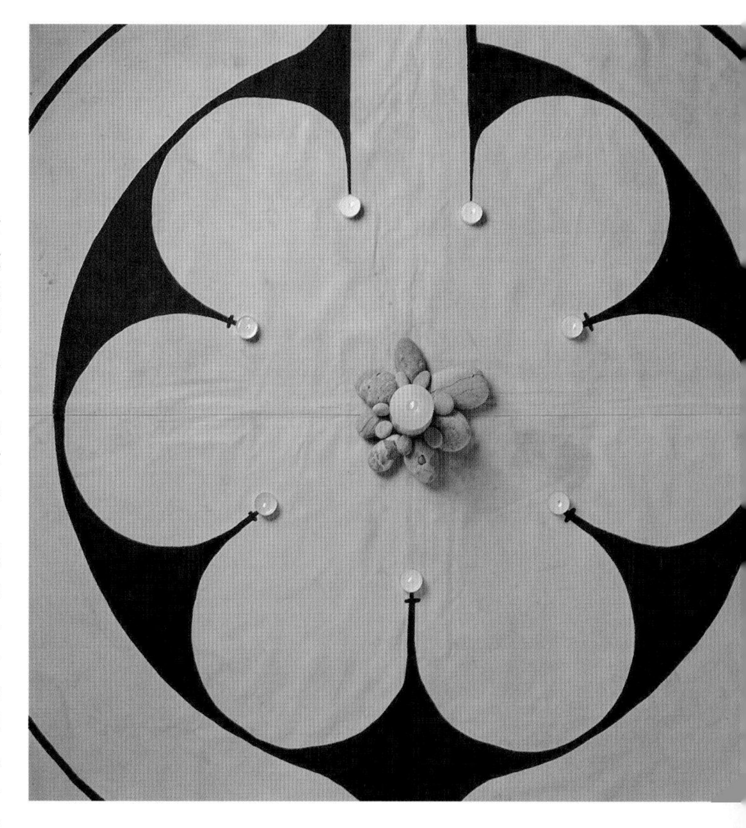

The resting place

After short stretches of pathway within each quarter of the Chartres labyrinth, you tread two very long semicircular sweeps near its outer edge. Although it appears that you are far away from the center, you will suddenly find yourself beside the straight entry path, heading directly for the center, completing the right-hand branch of the tree of life before you enter. The heart of the labyrinth is the goal or destination of your journey, but it is also a place where you can rest before completing your journey and making your way out.

The center space is contained within an open and empty circle, where you can stop moving; here you can rest, breathe, and be still. Pressed against the circumference of this open, circular space are six rounded petal shapes denoting harmony and balance. There are also six points in a circle. These are equidistant and form two triangles, one pointing up to the heavens, representing fire and the masculine, the other, pointing down to earth, water, and the feminine. Held in balance as you stand inside this configuration of six, you can receive a blessing through your crown or your feet. It may be the gift of a word, a feeling, or just stillness. Open your mind to the experience.

In a classical labyrinth the center is a smaller, open U-shaped space, where you can rest and take in inspiration, just like in the Chartres design. Indeed, the center of any design is a place where something new can take root and blossom, where you can let light into the center of your heart. Notice what you may usually be too rushed to see; ask a question you are normally too afraid to ask. It may be a place to express a hidden beauty, joy, or grief. Emptied of distraction, you now have the opportunity to be filled.

I have seen many things happen in the center: a traumatized woman curling up in a blanket and lying there for a long time, receiving the healing energy of a

At the center I met Pele, the Hawaiian Goddess of the volcano, who gave me fire, warmth, spirit, and inspiration, which I carried in my hands as she lead me out into the world again.

...the stillness at the heart of the labyrinth gains power and meaning from the twists and turns that precede it, which must be made first. Likewise, I know with a greater certainty that my experiences of wholeness and calm, when they come, are enriched by the convoluted business of everyday life.

Arriving at the center was a totally different energy. There were six of us there and it was very welcoming and supportive. I was aware of my feet on the ground but nothing else of me felt to exist. I was connected to a higher source.

The connection with something very powerful when I stepped right into the center took me by surprise. I wish I had stayed longer.

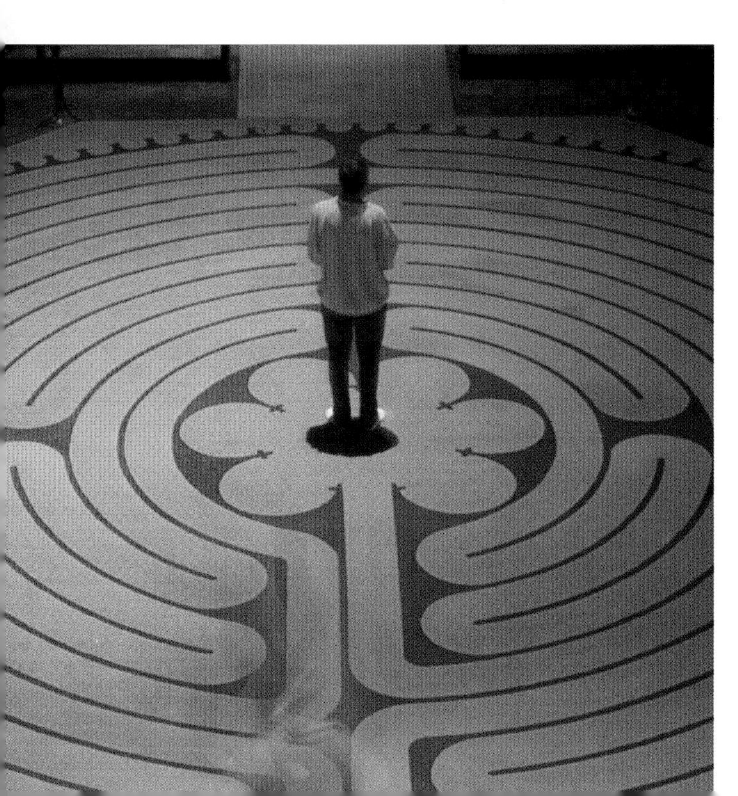

dance around the circumference of the labyrinth; a man and a woman celebrating their love with a little joyous jive sequence; school children dancing a flower dance; a woman weeping. Once I stood in the center with a prisoner at Brixton Prison and felt immensely strong and rooted, as if we were two standing stones in a stone circle.

The legend and the rose

Two images throw light on what can happen at the heart of the labyrinth. The first is of Theseus killing the Minotaur in the center (see p. 32), the legend that has been linked to the labyrinth for centuries. (This scene used to be depicted on a metal plaque in the central space of the Chartres labyrinth before it was removed in 1793 to make cannon.) With this in mind, the center becomes a place where a long-endured struggle can cease, where you can face what you most fear and dare to do the most difficult thing.

The second image glows in the darkness above the west door of Chartres Cathedral. It is the translucent, 12-petaled rose window, which has similar proportions to the labyrinth and would fit over it almost perfectly if the window could be folded down on top (see p. 39). As the light of the rose window falls on to the labyrinth below, the earthly journey is transformed with radiance and beauty. The feminine, represented by the rose, is united with the masculine in the form of Christ seated in judgment in the center of the window. His hands open wide on either side showing his wounds. In the Christian story, after suffering death, he returns, a living person, to his friends. He shows them his wounds saying, "Peace be with you." Hope and joy are thus born in the heart of the labyrinth, and the space opens like a flower, just like the rose in the heart of the window.

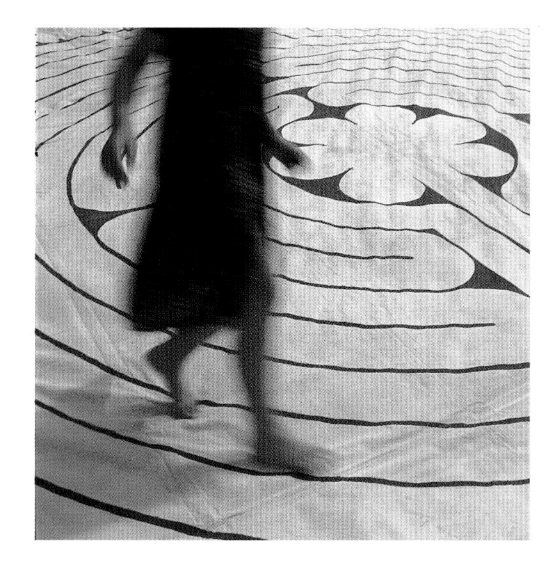

Coming out of the labyrinth I felt released into untrammeled life. I walked on the old stones of the floor, with the three blue windows and the rose window like a crown above me. It was a beautiful space. I was roaming free.

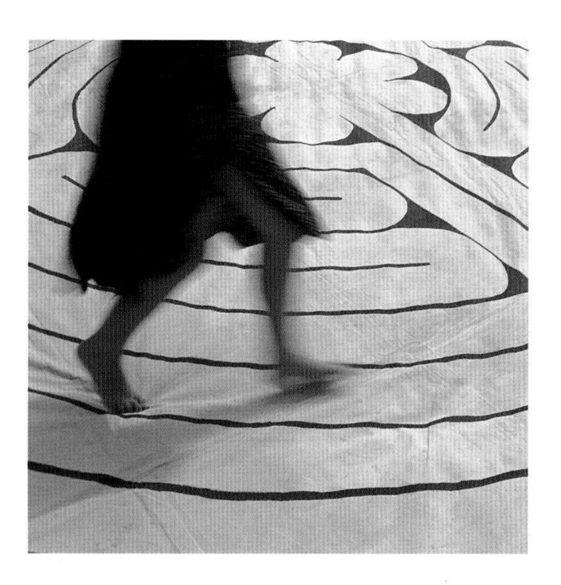

On the way out I felt desolate...I cried and felt utterly alone...As I moved toward the end my mood lightened and I wanted to speed up. I wanted to discharge a feeling of weight and seriousness. I felt very energized and enlivened after the labyrinth walk.

Journeying out

When you feel ready to leave the center, give thanks for whatever you have found or received there and begin your journey out again, following the same path you took on the way in. Let all the energy that has been coiled up in one direction be unwound and released. You may find that you feel faster, lighter, and funnier than you did on the way in. I remember one man saying he felt the center rise up before him like the top of a hill or tor. In the same way you may feel your journey out will be a release from any burdens you brought in with you. According to the legend, you now have the thread given by Ariadne to Theseus in your hand. You are connected and safe, and will find your way out easily to freedom and new life.

At this point small candles placed in the center previously can be lit and carried out through the labyrinth and into the world. If you have arranged

Treading the labyrinth for the first time was difficult for me—it felt like I was re-entering my mother's womb, and I could only feel intense grief. Coming out was a relief.... Treading the original labyrinth in Chartres Cathedral was a much more peaceful experience, deeply spiritual and connecting with the earth.

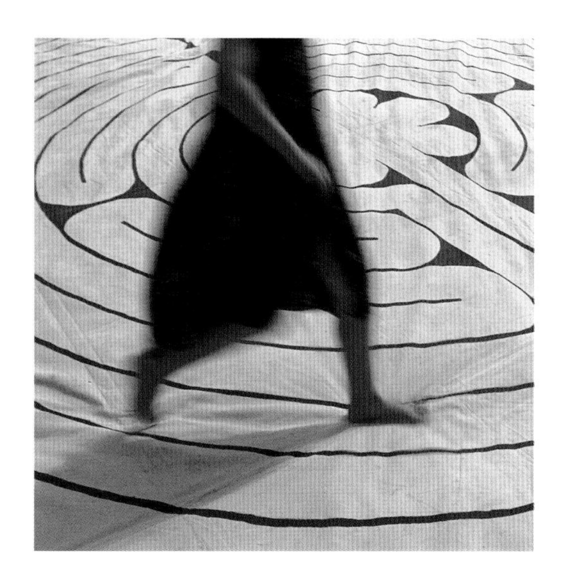

I could have run, cartwheeled, stamped, and shouted. For me the labyrinth is a re-energizer, a reminder of life, love, and giving.

multicolored ribbons at the center of the labyrinth, pilgrims can now choose one and weave it into a necklace or belt as a symbol of their journey and a reminder of Ariadne's thread (see p. 77). Alternatively, if you planned to celebrate a Christian Mass and placed offertory gifts of bread and wine at the center of the labyrinth, these can now be brought out by the participants and placed on the altar to be consecrated.

When you reach the exit, pause, give thanks, and rest. If you are using a canvas labyrinth, sit on one of the four corners to collect yourself; if you are on a turf labyrinth, sit on the grass, close your eyes, and breathe in the smells of nature around you. You may feel you need to express your journey in words or with images on paper or want to share your experience with another pilgrim. Perhaps you will want to sit quietly; perhaps you feel like running or somersaulting with joy.

Journeying together

In the Western tradition of the hero's or heroine's journey, we make the labyrinth pilgrimage alone. However, there is another tradition from Greece of dancing into the labyrinth as a linked-up chain of people to haunting music. You may wish to explore this after you have made your individual journey on the labyrinth as it provides a good contrast and will enrich your experience of treading labyrinths: while individual journeys tend to be introspective, a group journey will give you a strong sense of community and solidarity as you rock together on the path to the heart of the labyrinth.

The Sacred Circle Dance most often associated with the labyrinth is called *Tsakonikos*, meaning "from Tsakonia," a town in the Peloponnese. It is closely connected with the labyrinth and *Geranos*, the Crane Dance that Ariadne is said to have taught Theseus on the island of Naxos after their escape from Crete (see p. 32). You can learn how to perform this dance on pp. 72–73. The music to accompany it is simple and published alongside, although pre-recorded versions are also available (see Resources).

Before you begin, there are a number of considerations that you should bear in mind (right) to ensure a smooth journey. Try to practice the dance off the labyrinth first to get a feel for the group's rhythm.

Whether you tread the labyrinth on your own or with others as part of a group, each person's experience is different. This chapter suggests how you can make the journey to the center of the labyrinth and out again. Use any of the ideas that immediately appeal to you and entrust yourself to the journey. Chapter Four offers guidelines on how to ground yourself after your experience on the labyrinth and re-enter everyday life.

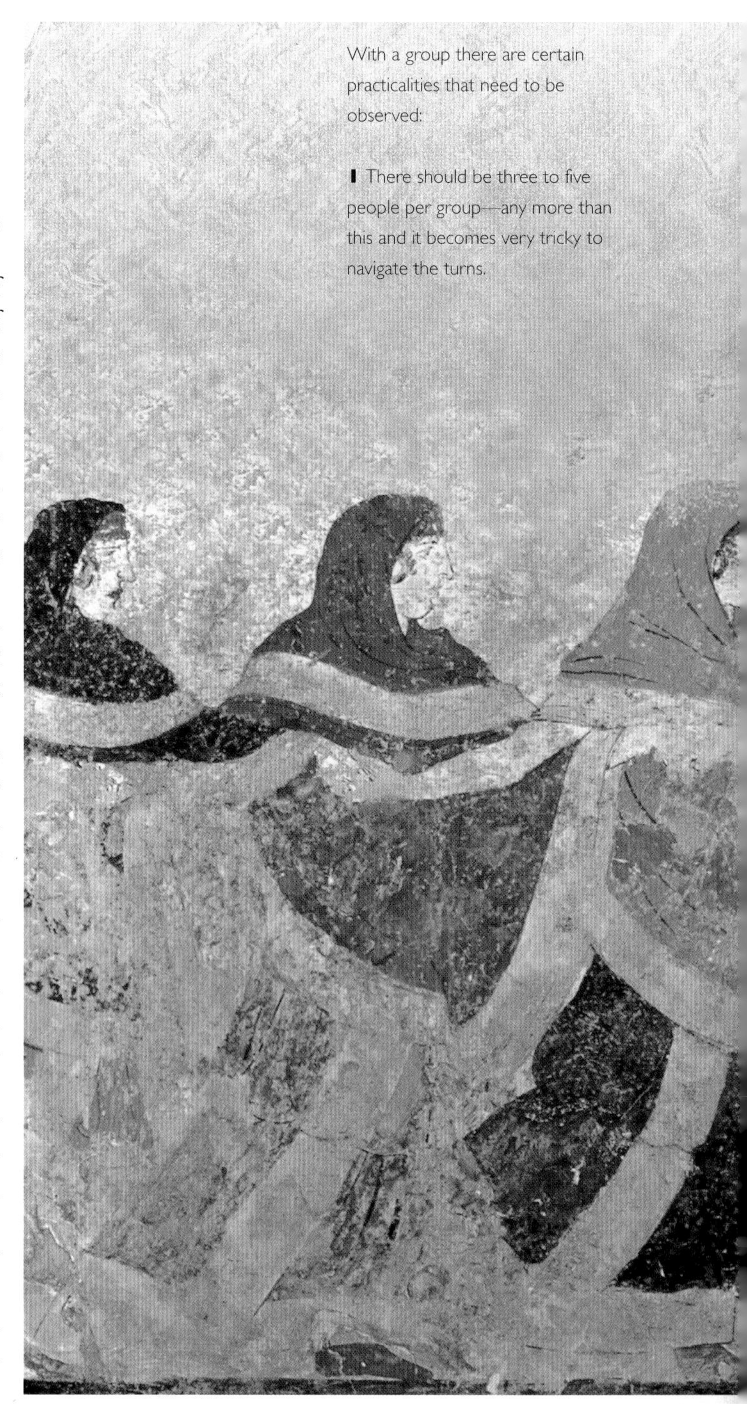

With a group there are certain practicalities that need to be observed:

- There should be three to five people per group—any more than this and it becomes very tricky to navigate the turns.

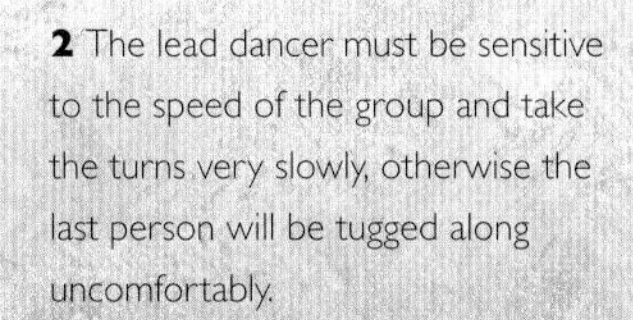

2 The lead dancer must be sensitive to the speed of the group and take the turns very slowly, otherwise the last person will be tugged along uncomfortably.

3 The proper dance handhold for *Tsakonikos* (see p. 72) is difficult to sustain on the turns, so you can adapt it to a loose handhold. This can be broken momentarily as the chain eases around a corner.

4 If there is only one group on the labyrinth, you can join up in a circle at the center for a while, and then dance back out. If there are two or three groups, it is more practical if the first one, after spending time at the center, weaves out across the pathways, carefully avoiding the other groups, and continues to dance around the circumference of the labyrinth, holding the journeys of those still inside.

5 The group *Tsakonikos* experience is very mesmeric because of the repetition of simple steps to the powerful music (see pp. 72–72) and rhythmic swaying of the group.

You can try other Greek, classical or modern music that has a continuous flow. *A Pilgrim's Dance* choreographed to the music of Pachelbel's *Canon*, consisting of three steps forwards, and one sway back, also works well on the labyrinth.

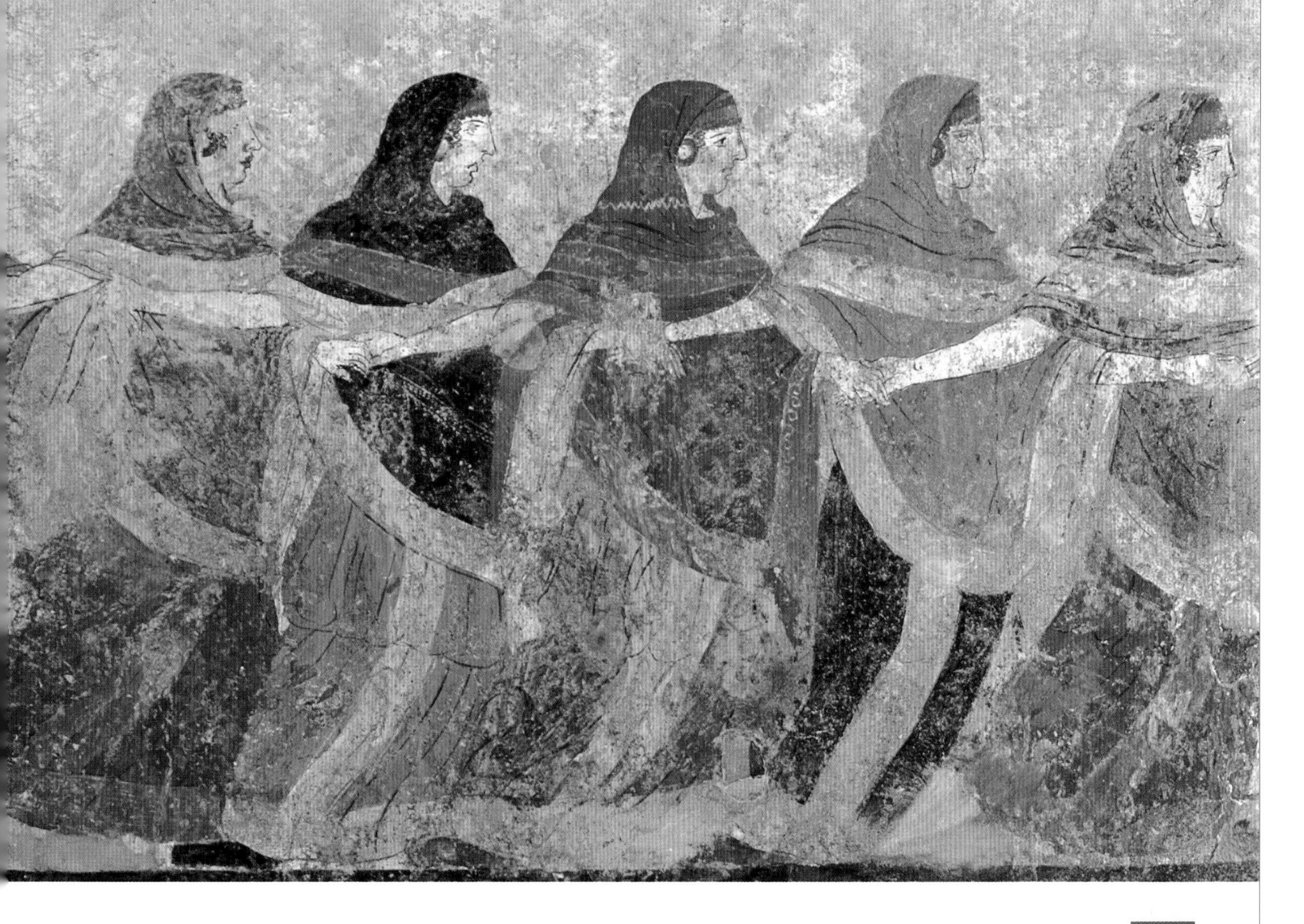

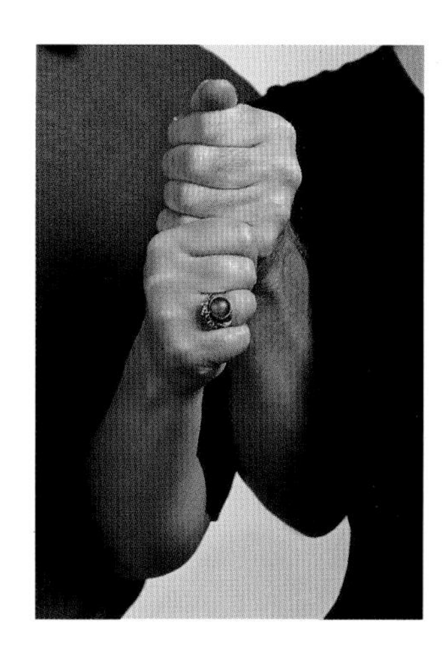

Link your right elbow over your neighbor's left and extend your right thumb to be held by the hand of the dancer on your right. If you find it difficult to navigate the turns with this grip, just hold each other's hands with your arms held close to your bodies.

The Crane Dance

With its simple tune and swaying steps, *Tsakonikos* is a mesmerizing dance that you perform in a close chain of people, ideal for weaving in and out of the spirals of the labyrinth. Remember to keep your groups small, otherwise you will not be able to navigate the labyrinth's turns. The handhold (right) is said to be symbolic of carrying candles through the labyrinth, although it also carries a more obvious sexual meaning, which ties it in with the mating dance of the crane bird and the themes of fertility and new life.

Move sideways to the right with your feet pointing at a 45 degree angle to the right, but keep your torso facing straight ahead. This creates a twist in the hips. The rhythm of the music is 5/4, which you may find difficult to follow. Try counting it as 1, 2, 3, 4, pause.

A Repeat A four times. This sequence corresponds to the notes of one bar of tune A (in beat 3 the two quavers are one action). Begin with your feet together.

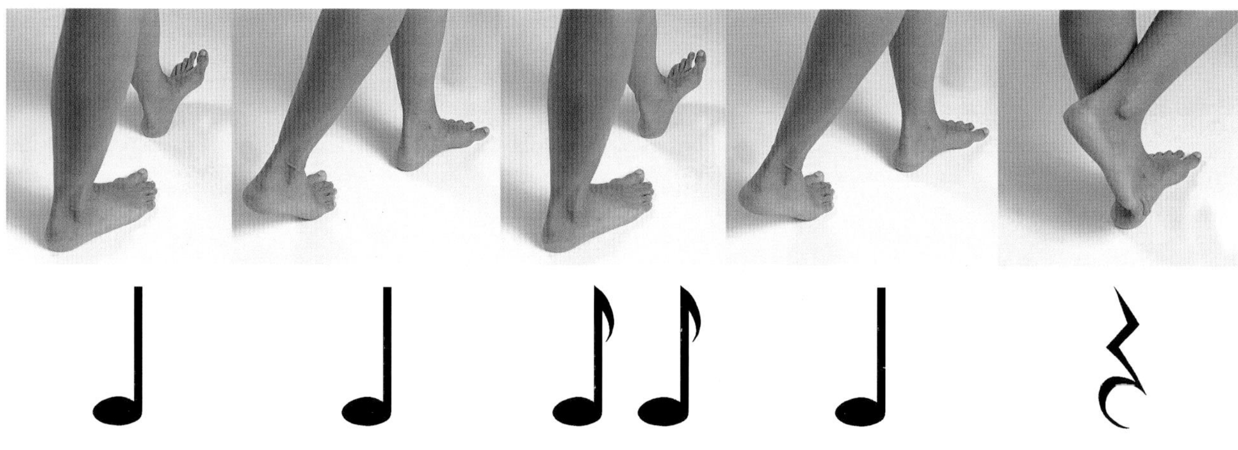

Beat 1 Step backwards on to your right foot in a rocking movement, placing it behind your left.

Beat 2 Rock forwards on to your left foot, crossing it in front of your right.

Beat 3 Rock back on to your right foot, placing it behind your left in a small step to the right.

Beat 4 Rock forwards again on your left foot, crossing it in front of your right.

Beat 5 (This beat is silent.) Tap your right toe lightly behind the heel of the left foot and start the sequence again.

tune A

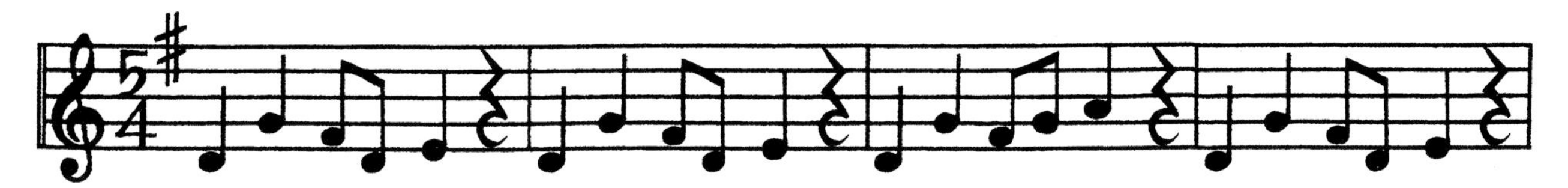

tune B

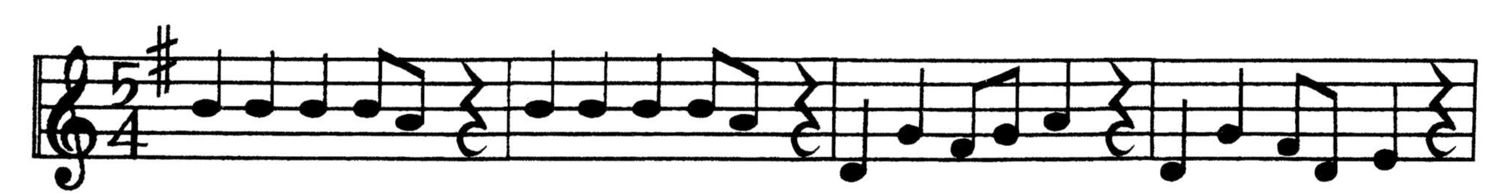

B Repeat this part four times as in A. Tune B varies, so beats 3 and 4 below correspond either to one quaver or one crochet, although the steps are the same.

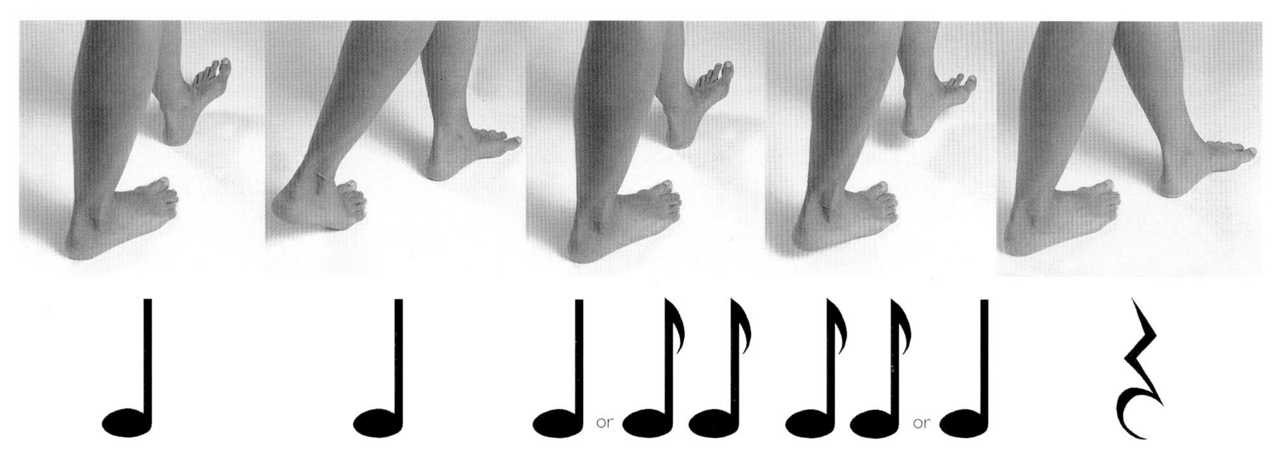

Beat 1 Step backwards on to your right foot in a rocking movement, placing it behind your left.

Beat 2 Rock forwards on to your left foot, crossing it in front of your right.

Beat 3 Rock back on to your right foot, placing it behind your left in a small step to the right.

Beat 4 Make a tiny hop on the right foot as you lift the left foot off the ground, crossing it over and in front of the right.

Beat 5 (This beat is silent.) Place the left foot down and in front of the right foot.

4

GROUNDING IN THE PRESENT

The world is clean—washed by the rain,
fresh and new, smelling of
damp earth, green grass and spring;
and I feel as if life were beginning
again for me, that like the
willows, I have renewed my bones
with fledgling leaves. My face
turned upward to welcome the rain;
and I, for all my years, am newly born,
seeing the world with wondering eyes.
Marla Visser

When you have completed your journey through the labyrinth, you may feel deeply moved or re-energized by your experience. Whatever you have found on the labyrinth, you need to ground yourself, find your ordinary feet again and give thanks for what you have received. In Chapter Two you prepared the ground, awakening the energies of the labyrinth in space, among people and in time. You now need to close down each dimension in turn, only this time in reverse order.

The dimension of time helped to anchor the labyrinth in its surroundings, and in the same way it will bring you back to the present. Equally, the movement of people on and around the labyrinth played an important part in waking the energies of both labyrinth and pilgrims, which now have to be earthed before you dismantle the area you used. Attention to the third dimension, space, played an important part in preparing the labyrinth for use, especially when placing a portable one either indoors or outdoors. Full of thanksgiving, you can now dismantle it, and let the space sink back into its ordinary state again.

How you choose to ground yourself will depend largely on how you prepared each dimension before you walked the labyrinth and what you experienced on its path. Be sensitive to your mood and that of any other pilgrims who may be with you. Whatever you decide to do, make sure that you close down all three dimensions so that you are fully protected in everyday space and time.

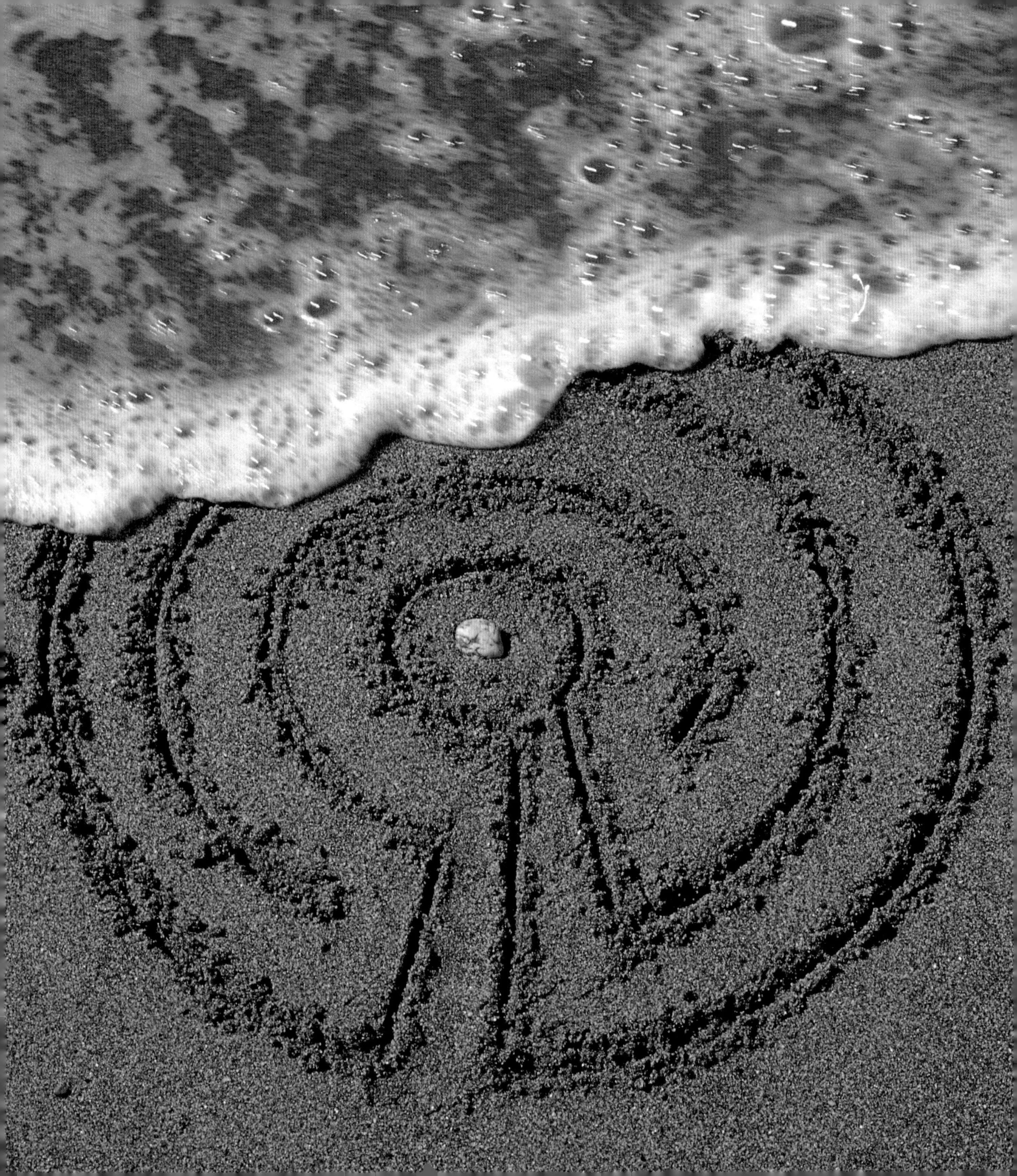

Closing the labyrinth in time

Whether you have journeyed alone or in a group there are a number of ways you can close the ritual space of a labyrinth in time. It is often helpful to revisit the season you explored before you stepped on to the labyrinth in Chapter Two or to remember the people from the past you called on to guide you through it. To do this you can dance the "Cycle of the Year" again (see p. 54), tracing the year's cycle over your body.

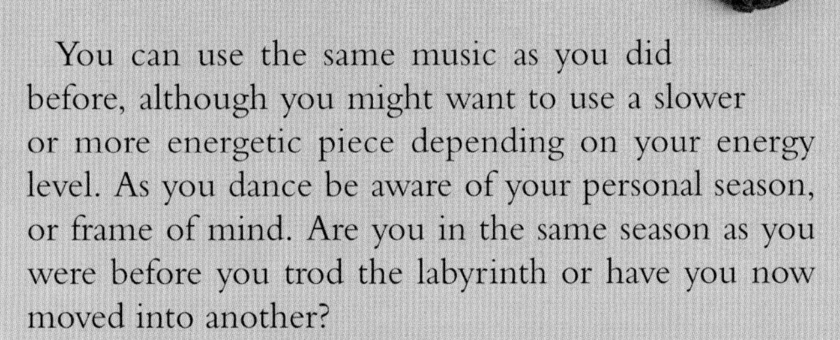

You can use the same music as you did before, although you might want to use a slower or more energetic piece depending on your energy level. As you dance be aware of your personal season, or frame of mind. Are you in the same season as you were before you trod the labyrinth or have you now moved into another?

If you prepared a seasonal altar, you can now consume any food or drink you arranged on it, such as apples for Halloween, milk for Candlemas, eggs for Easter, or bread for autumn. If you have a favorite poem read it out loud to help you meditate on the season you have honored. Does the mood of the poem reflect the season of your soul? Alternatively, if you asked figures from the past to help you walk the labyrinth, you can now thank these either by calling out their names or saying them silently in your mind. Perhaps you will want them to protect you in ordinary space as well. In the same way you can also thank any guardians or elders that you called into the space when you were preparing the ground.

Ariadne's thread

If you have a portable labyrinth and want to remember the people who have walked it or the places it has visited, you can make an Ariadne memory thread. You need a ball of brightly colored string, on to which you can attach tags or mementos that are symbolic of your journey. Twine your Ariadne's thread around a cylinder to store it in between each labyrinth event. When you close down the labyrinth in time, you can read out the names of people and the places visited to link the labyrinth with time present, thereby creating a sense of continuity and community. The thread also resonates with the myth of Theseus and the Minotaur (see p. 32) and the labyrinth at Knossos, which connects your recent journey on the labyrinth with time past.

Two weeks on [after treading the labyrinth] and I feel clearer—more confident and less stressed. A transformation that friends have commented on.

The time [I] spent walking the labyrinth at Chartres gave me a feeling of being enfolded, cradled, acknowledged, and accepted for what I am and the part I play in the whole.

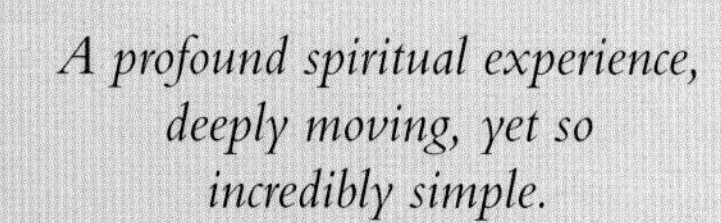

A profound spiritual experience, deeply moving, yet so incredibly simple.

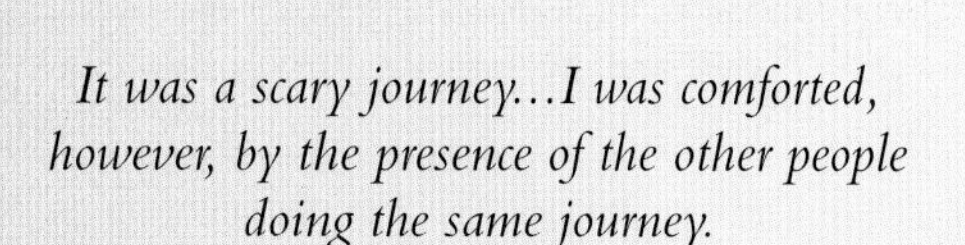

It was a scary journey...I was comforted, however, by the presence of the other people doing the same journey.

You had to concentrate hard. I was aware that I rush at things while other people were much more deliberate—was this a message? A centering experience.

Human energy to close the space

This is my play's last scene,
here heavens appoint
My pilgrimage's last mile.
John Donne

Just as you used your energies to quicken those of the space, so too do you need to use human movement to close the labyrinth. One way you can do this is by paying attention to your breathing. If you are alone and indoors, stand quietly and breathe deeply into your center, which is located just below your navel. Release your breath, sending it down into the earth. Repeat about ten times and enjoy the feeling of relaxation that washes over your body.

Use your hands to circle up and receive the breath, exhaling as your hands pass straight down from your head to your root and over your torso. This deepens your breathing and roots you to the earth. You might like to burn your favorite incense or essential oils to help you focus on your breathing. Lavender is good for calming and stabilizing your energies, while grapefruit will refresh and revive your spirits. Cedarwood can also help to restore a sense of spiritual certainty and strengthen your resolve.

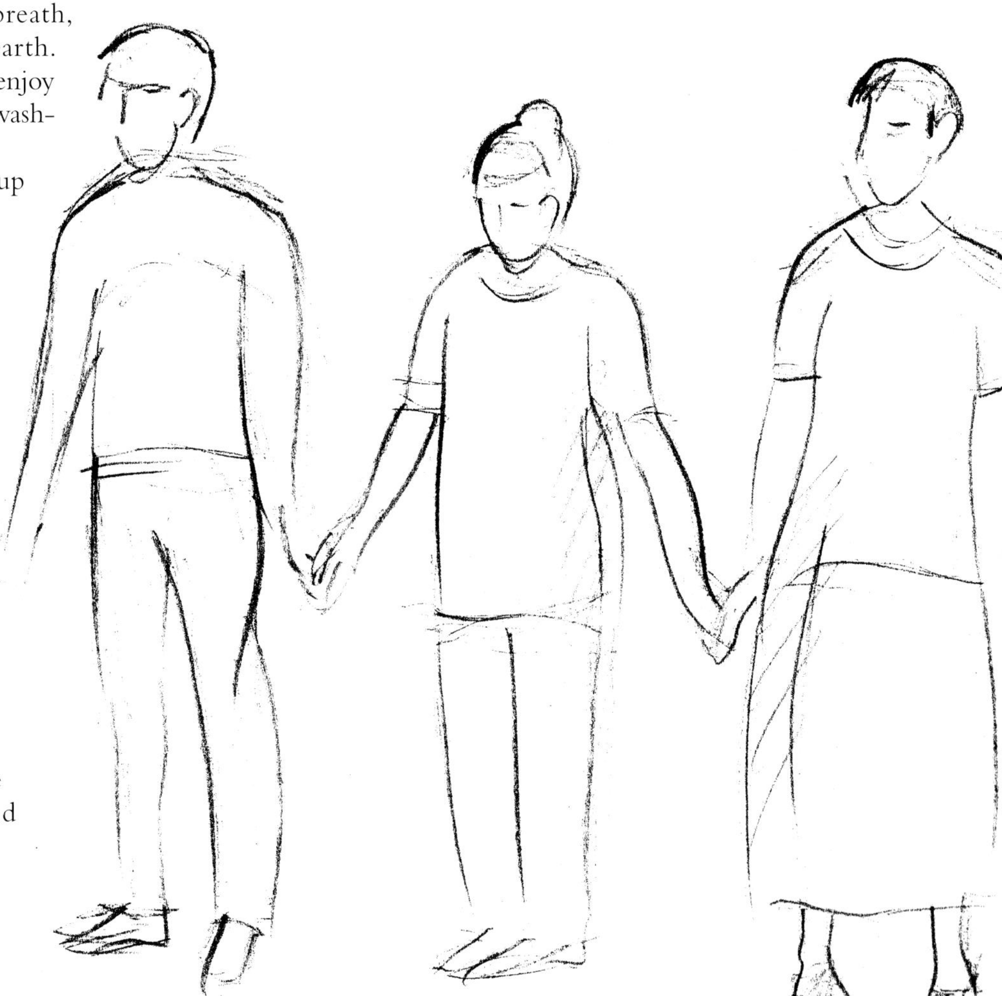

Grounding group energies

If you are performing the breathing exercise in a big group, you can all stand around the perimeter of the labyrinth. Breathe and sway to some gentle music before you begin. Alternatively, come close together in a circle on the labyrinth, with your hands hooked behind each other and holding the waists of the pilgrims beside you. Be still for a moment. Standing in this way with a supportive touch on the lower spine is immensely comforting and grounding. You can also join in a dance to close the space, using one of the basic shapes outlined in Chapter Two, namely the circle, the spiral or the horseshoe. Match the mood of the place and people with the pace and music you play—quiet, meditative music may be appropriate or perhaps you will need something rhythmic and joyful. At the end of the dance stand still in the quiet for a few moments and breathe in deeply.

Finally, you may wish to ground yourself with a visualization technique to close and protect the chakra system of the body (see p. 60). You can imagine each chakra has petals, which you can close gently at the root of the torso, the sacral area just below the navel, the solar plexus, the heart, the throat, the brow, and the crown of the head. At each chakra point you can visualize drawing over it a ring of light containing a cross of light. This will protect you from being too vulnerable as you re-enter ordinary life.

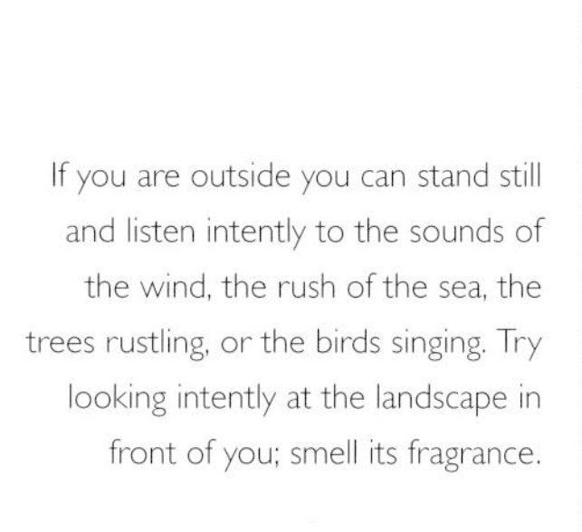

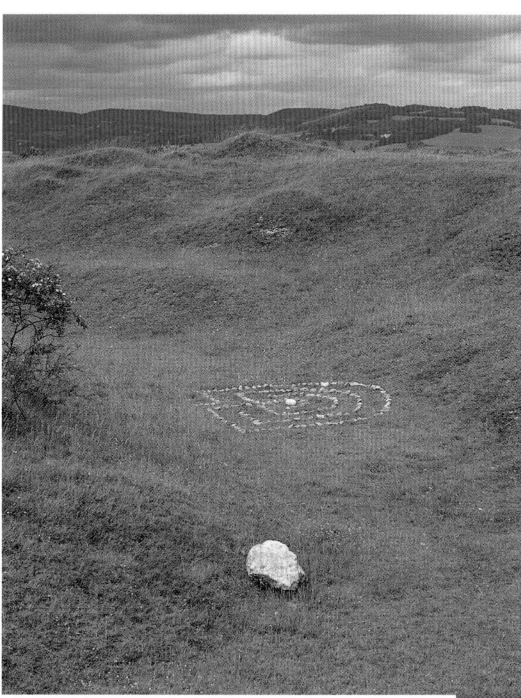

If you are outside you can stand still and listen intently to the sounds of the wind, the rush of the sea, the trees rustling, or the birds singing. Try looking intently at the landscape in front of you; smell its fragrance.

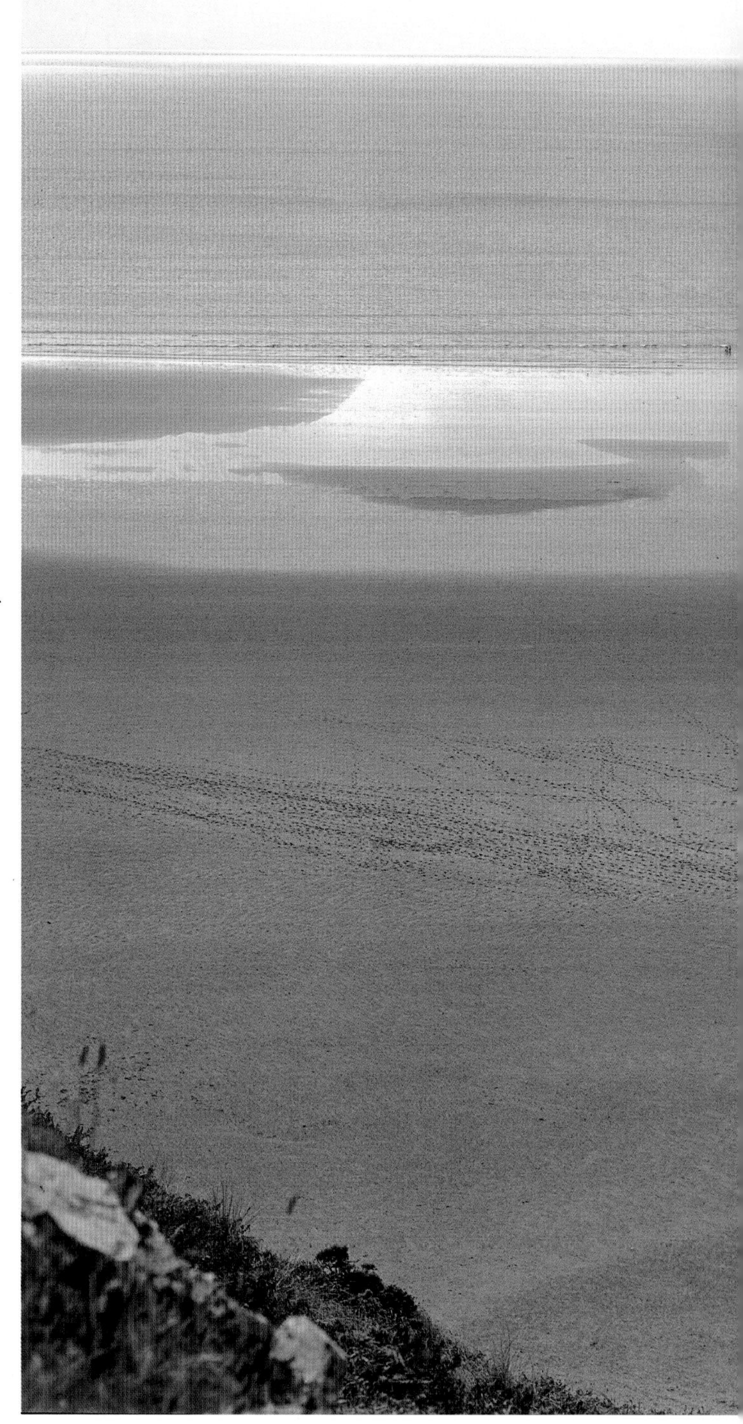

Closing the ritual space

Once you have grounded your energy, the labyrinth space can be closed. If you are alone and outdoors on a turf or beach labyrinth, you can walk around it, pausing at each corner to give thanks. If you are indoors with a small finger labyrinth, you can give thanks and pause, holding your hands over your heart before extinguishing the candles. Watch the smoke curl up and dissolve into the air. Wherever you are, open your hands and send out the energy of your journey into the world.

If you have been walking the labyrinth as part of a group, stand around it in a circle holding hands. Any candles you used to simulate fire energy (see pp. 44–46) and bring the space to life can now be snuffed out, and the energy commended to the air. If you positioned a candle on each of the labyrinth's four axes, ask four individuals to return them one by one to the rose center. With each candle the point of the compass and its element can be named, and the associated archangel thanked for blessings given. Alternatively, if you used the Chartres design and placed night lights in each of the lunations (see p. 96), everybody can stand around the labyrinth and blow them out together. Each pilgrim can take two or three away with them as a reminder of their journey.

Before you blow out the candles you might find it helpful to name out loud one gift you received on your labyrinth journey. The group can then hold it in consciousness for a moment. Thank the space, perhaps with a reading, poem, or prayer, and blow out the four candles together, sending the energy and light of the labyrinth and your dancing into the world, wherever it may be needed.

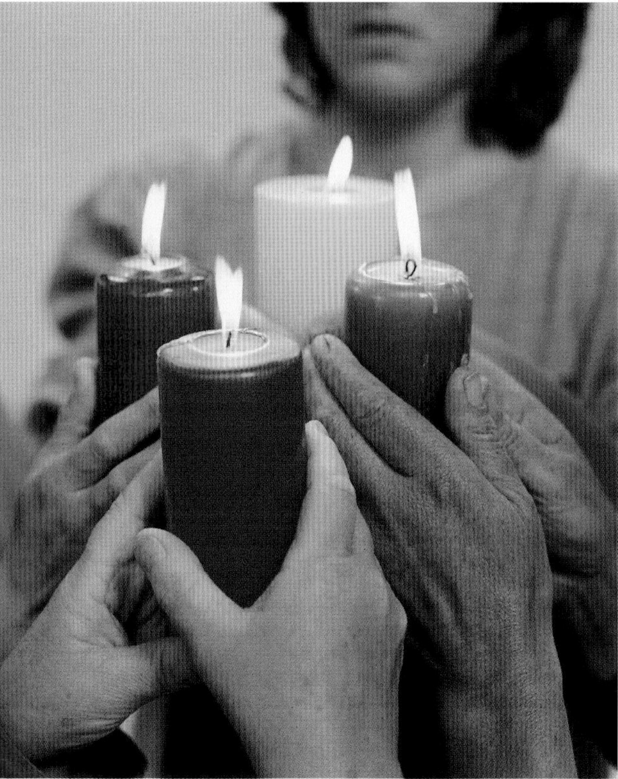

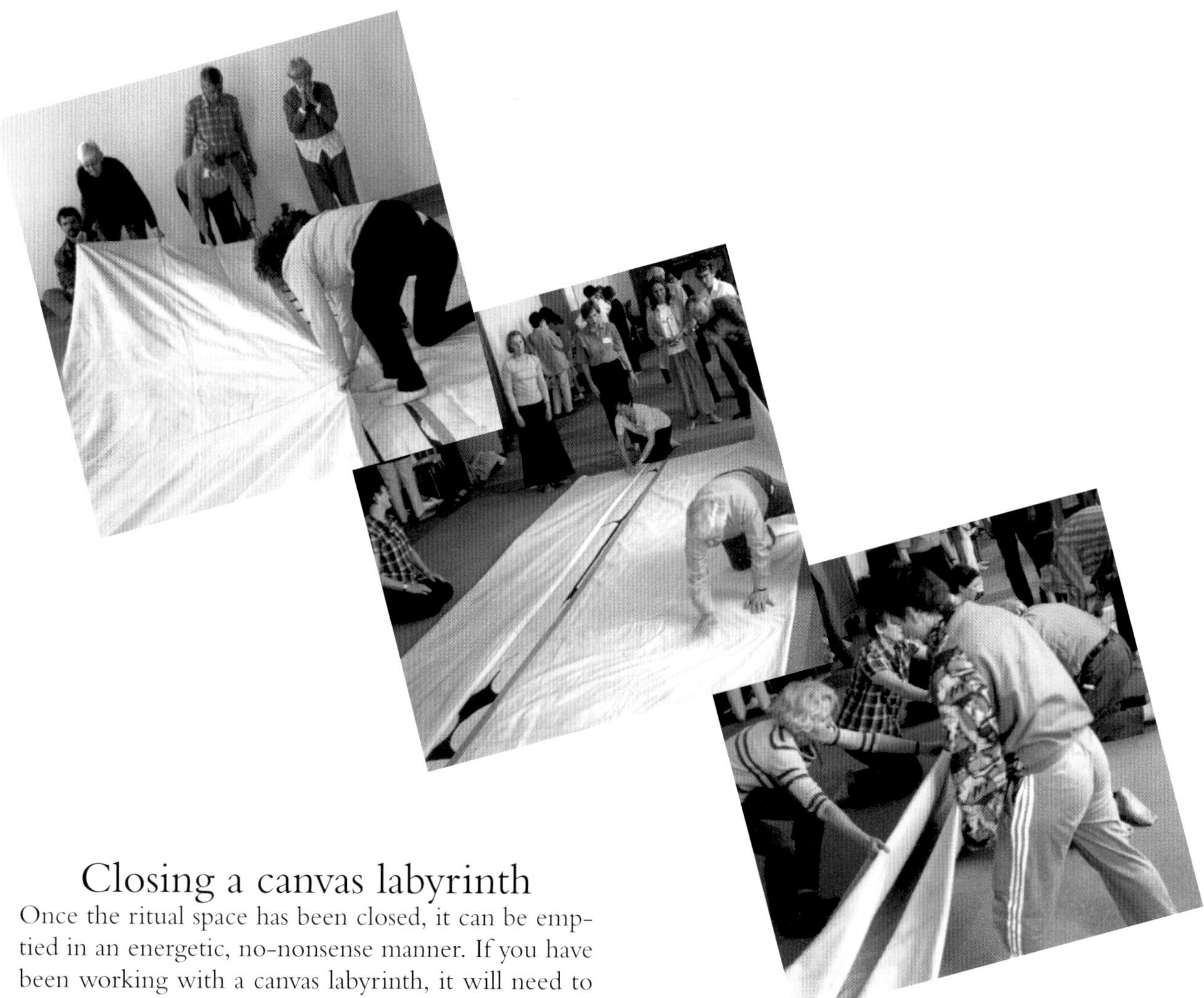

Closing a canvas labyrinth

Once the ritual space has been closed, it can be emptied in an energetic, no-nonsense manner. If you have been working with a canvas labyrinth, it will need to be packed up and prepared for its next destination, just like a Bedouin tent or a Native American tepee has to be dismantled before journeying on.

Before you do this, you can give the whole surface of the canvas a good sweep with a stiff broom—rhythmic strokes make a pleasant scraping music that helps to bring you back to the here and now. The familiar sounds of matter interacting with matter, of bristle brushing canvas, are full of solace and simple joy. This will ensure that it is clean and fresh for the next destination. If the canvas has been outside and is damp or wet from condensation or rain, it will need special attention to ensure it dries properly. Make sure you lay it out in a hall or large space as soon as possible so it can dry out. The canvas may obtain an attractive antique patina effect as a result.

Folding up the canvas with precision can also help to ground the individual in the present and will give each pilgrim a sense of community, as it requires group cooperation. It also shows respect for the space

Let us be united;
Let us speak in harmony;
Let our minds apprehend alike.
Common be our prayer;
Common be the end of our assembly;
Common be our resolution;
Common be our deliberations.
Alike be our feelings;
Unified be our hearts;
Common be our intentions;
Perfect be our unity.
The Rig Veda

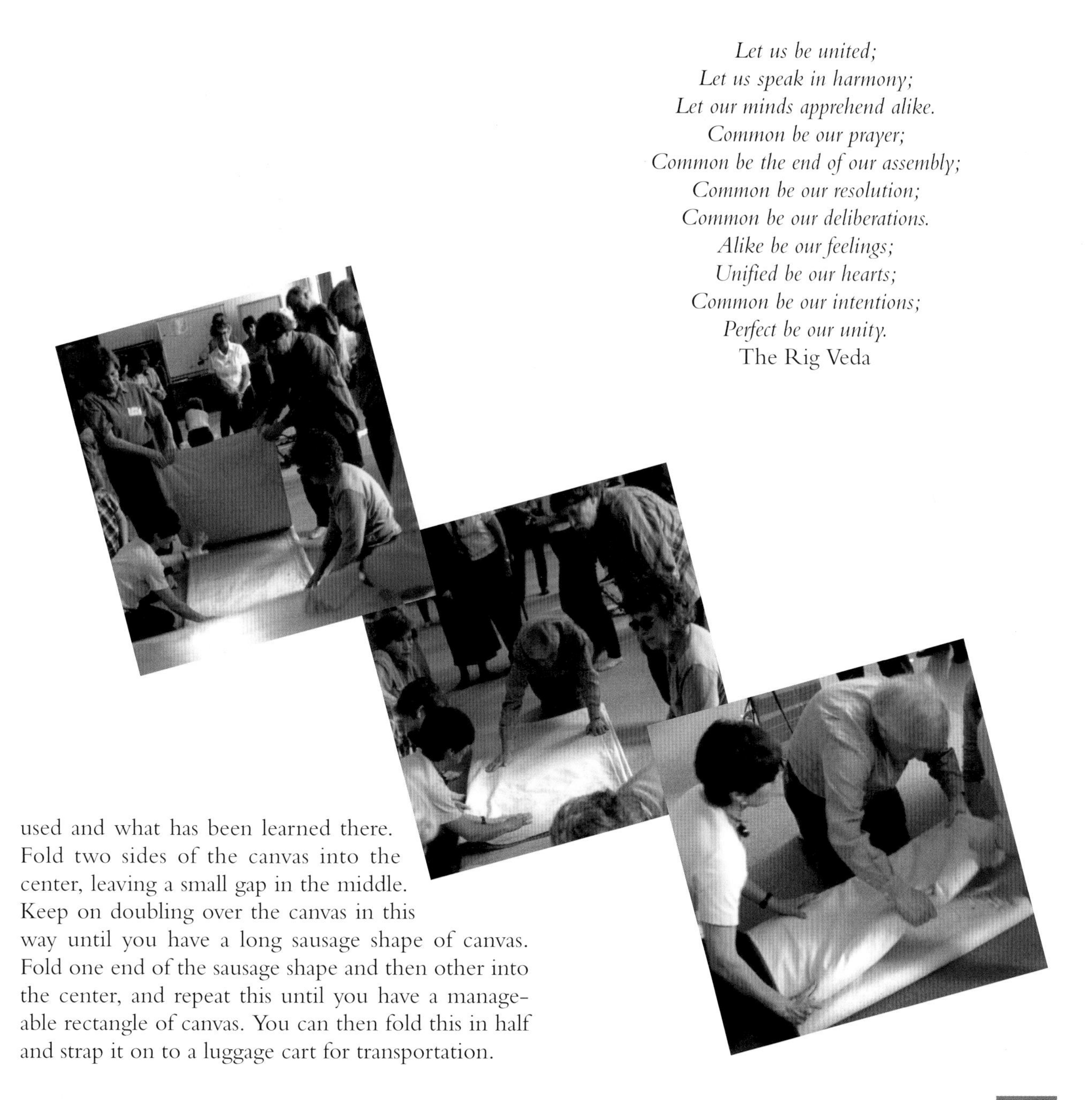

used and what has been learned there. Fold two sides of the canvas into the center, leaving a small gap in the middle. Keep on doubling over the canvas in this way until you have a long sausage shape of canvas. Fold one end of the sausage shape and then other into the center, and repeat this until you have a manageable rectangle of canvas. You can then fold this in half and strap it on to a luggage cart for transportation.

Leaving the space

When the labyrinth has been folded away, you can turn your attention to all the other things you used, such as candles or tape recorders, so you can leave the space tidy but not unchanged. Before leaving, if you are alone and outside, welcome in the night that will make it invisible to the human eye. With a labyrinth you have cut or drawn into a sandy beach, greet the incoming tide that will wash away the pathways. Commend a labyrinth you have chalked on to asphalt

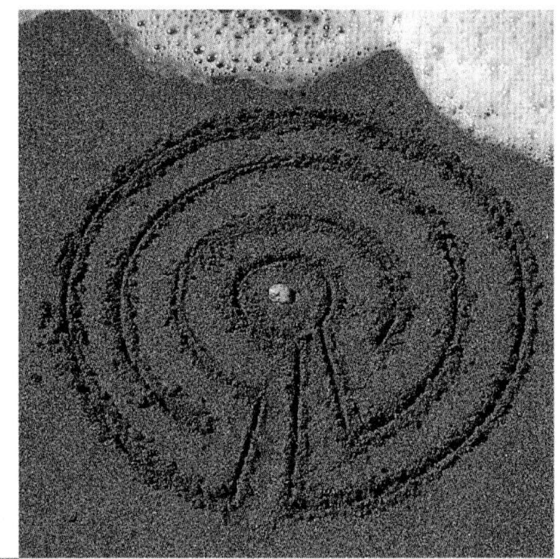

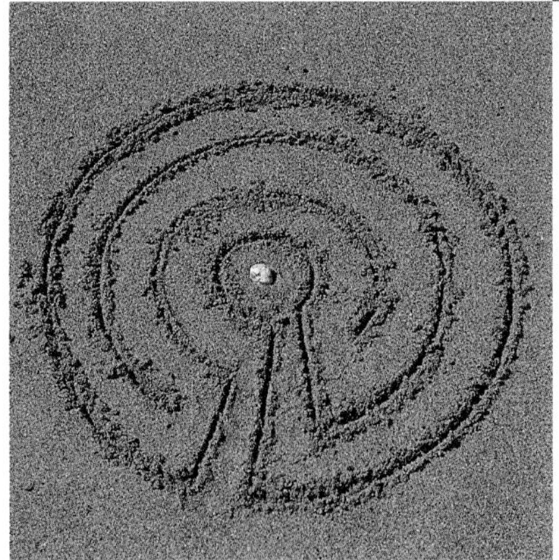

O our Father, the Sky, hear us and make us strong.
O our Mother, the Earth, hear us and give us support.
O Spirit of the East, send us your wisdom.
O Spirit of the South, may we tread your path of life.
O Spirit of the West, may be always be ready for the long journey.
O Spirit of the North, purify us with your cleansing winds.
Sioux prayer

to the feet and the rain that will gradually rub out the circuits. If you are indoors with a small labyrinth on paper, place it in a special envelope and pack it away. Remove any photographs, crystals, or flowers that you used to make an indoor space sacred, and open a window to let in fresh air to cleanse the space. You can then leave the room, closing the door behind you.

Now that you have closed down the labyrinth in time, among people, and in space, the circle of your journey on the labyrinth is complete. If you have found hidden emotions on your journey, continue to explore them away from the labyrinth in whatever way comes naturally to you. This may be in writing, painting, dancing, or conversation with others. Hold on to what you may have learned about yourself and enjoy the energy flowing through your body. In this way the labyrinth can become a pathway to healing your mind and body, for its coils offer you space to relax mentally and physically, and to meditate on your pathway through life. Too often we suppress our thoughts and emotions in the stresses of our daily routines and are too busy to eat properly or sleep long enough hours. Although our bodies can tolerate this initially, constant pressure can lead to depression or serious illness in later life. Treading the labyrinth gives you time to listen to yourself and your needs, as well as to replenish your energy levels. Not only will this encourage your physical health but it will also help you to lead a happier and more relaxed lifestyle.

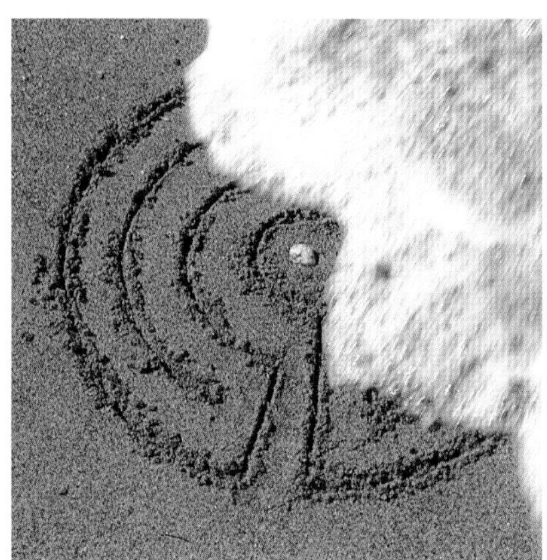

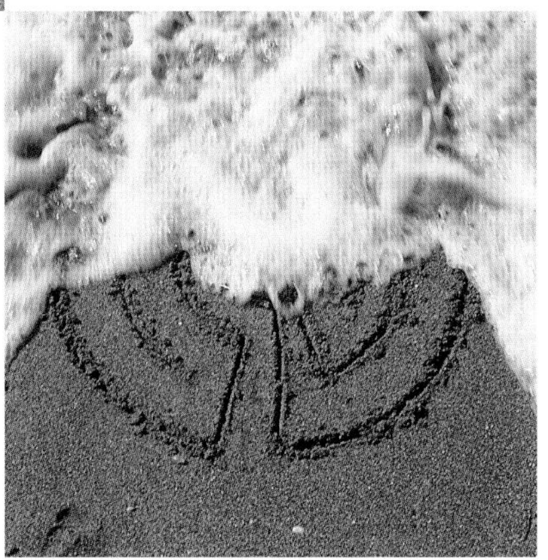

The great sea has set me in motion.
Set me adrift,
And I move as a weed in the river.

The arch of the sky
And mightiness of storms
Encompasses me,
And I am left
Trembling with joy.
Eskimo song

5

CREATING YOUR OWN LABYRINTH

A journey with labyrinths would be incomplete without learning how to create your own, so this chapter will look at some of the designs we have come across in the previous chapters. We will begin by studying the classical design in two forms, the simple three-circuit and the more elaborate seven-circuit. The easiest way to come to grips with the classical design is to draw it on paper and trace its path with a finger. You can then consider more ambitious projects, made with a variety of different materials, that are large enough to walk.

Once you have familiarized yourself with the classical design, you will probably want to develop ideas using the Chartres labyrinth. Although this design is quite complicated, there are some easy methods you can use to create temporary labyrinths with chalk on asphalt or with sticks on sand. These you can walk as described in Chapters Two to Four. However, you may like to make a precise copy of the Chartres labyrinth, so this chapter will also show you how to work out the exact dimensions of the Chartres design, which you can transfer on to the material of your choice, such as canvas.

If you do not have access to a large space to make a Chartres labyrinth or to unfold a canvas copy, then you can photocopy the design on p. 96 and paint the pathways with watercolors as another form of meditation. Alternatively, you can consult the Resources at the back of the book (see pp. 106–109) to find out about labyrinth organizations in your area and if there are any labyrinths you can walk near by. Certain organizations even supply ready-made canvas labyrinths, although these are quite expensive.

If you decide to make a labyrinth outside, remember to respect the surrounding environment. Don't, for example, remove stones permanently from beaches as this can encourage land erosion. Equally, if you are making a temporary labyrinth in a public place, ensure that you leave the space as you found it. Whatever kind of labyrinth you make, the most important thing is to enjoy it and to open your heart to your experience on its path.

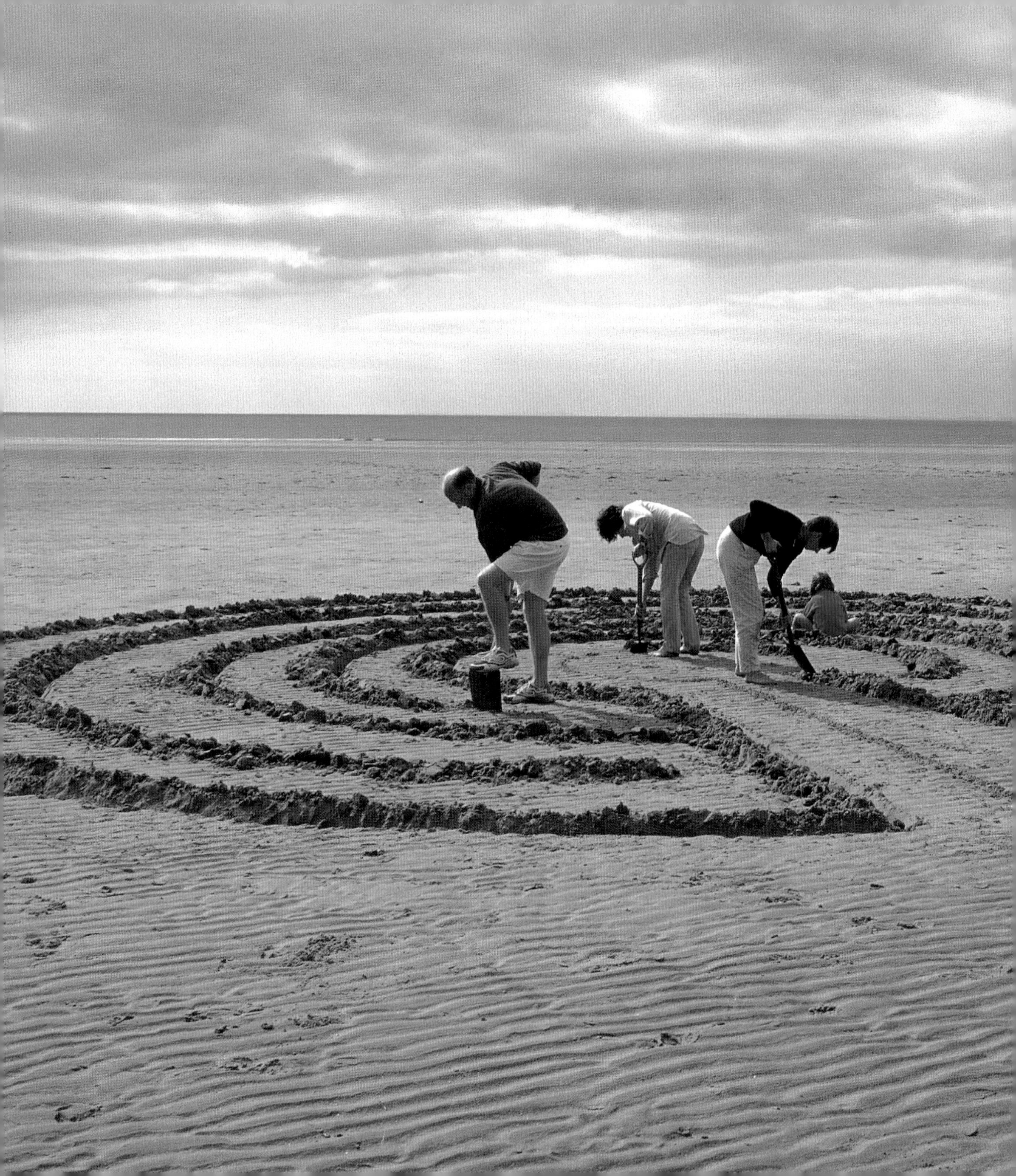

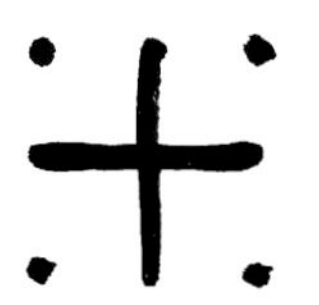

1 Draw a cross and mark a dot in each quadrant.

The three-path classical design

The best way to get to grips with labyrinth design is to draw one until it becomes automatic. You can create a labyrinth with its entrance lying either to the left or to the right of the design. To make a left-entry labyrinth connect the top of the initial cross you draw with the top right-hand dot of the quadrant (see right). For a right-entry labyrinth, the reverse is true: join the top of the cross with the top left-hand dot and draw from right to left.

To begin with, always return to the same side of the drawing to connect it with the other. When you are used to this method, you can vary this. Try drawing the first line from left to right, the second from right to left and so on. This method feels similar to walking the sweeping paths of a labyrinth. With either variation you will find that the movement becomes a growing spiral. Drawing labyrinths exercises left and right brain actions and tests hand–eye coordination.

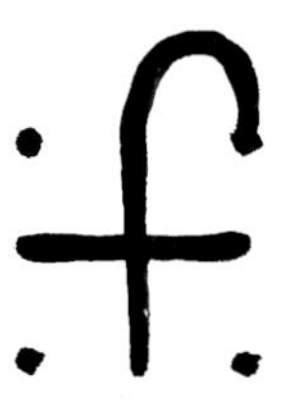

2 Connect the top of the cross with the top right-hand dot to form a crook shape.

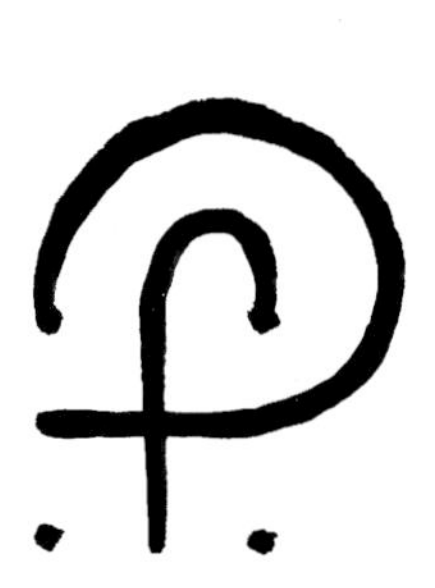

3 Return to the top left-hand dot and draw an arc to connect with the right side of the horizontal line.

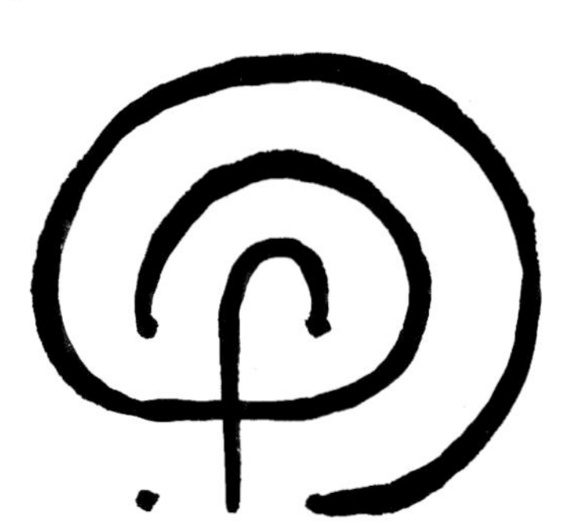

4 Now join the left side of the horizontal line in a broad sweep over the top to the lower right-hand dot.

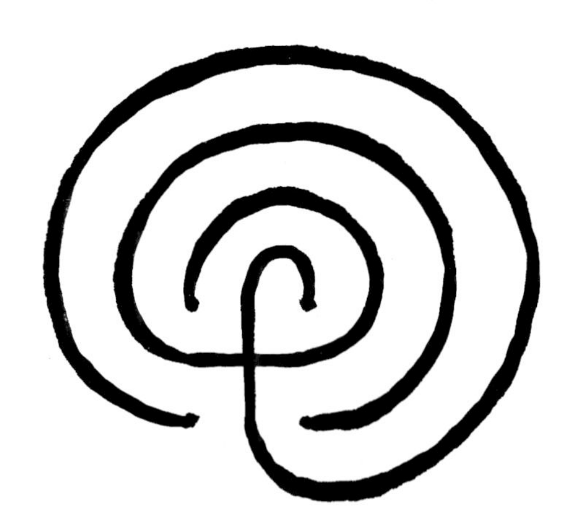

5 Lastly, connect the bottom left-hand dot all the way over the top and around to the bottom of the vertical axis.

The seven-path classical design

When you are familiar with the three-circuit classical labyrinth you can draw a seven-circuit labyrinth. It works on the same principles, only you add four corner angles between the crossed central axes and the dots. You can determine whether you get a left- or right-entry labyrinth by applying the three-circuit rules on p. 88. When you draw this design you will notice that the initial crossed lines are not directly in the center of the design. For this reason you need to begin your drawing about a third from the bottom of your space, as the emerging circuits need to expand into the top two thirds of the space. Practice this shape until it becomes automatic.

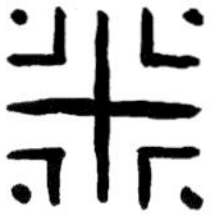

1 Draw a cross as you did for the three-circuit design, only this time draw a corner angle in each quadrant. Mark each of the four quadrants with a dot.

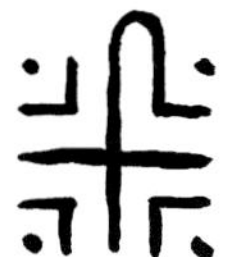

2 Connect the top of the cross with the vertical line of the top right-hand corner angle. This will form the center space of the labyrinth.

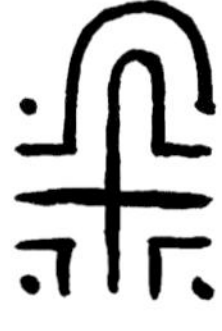

3 Next join the vertical line of the top left-hand corner angle with the top right-hand dot.

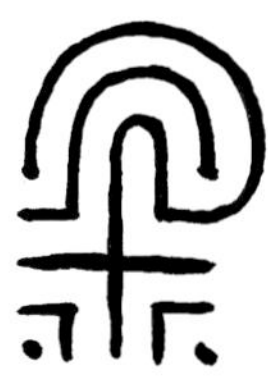

4 Return to the top left-hand dot and draw an arc to connect with the horizontal line of the top right-hand corner angle.

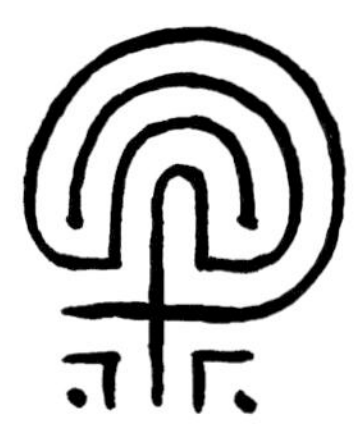

5 Join the horizontal line of the top left-hand corner angle in a broad sweep to the right horizontal arm of the cross.

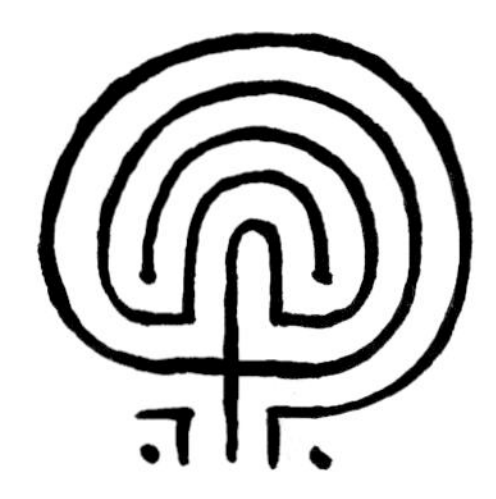

6 Now draw an arc from the left horizontal arm of the cross to the horizontal line of the lower right-hand corner angle.

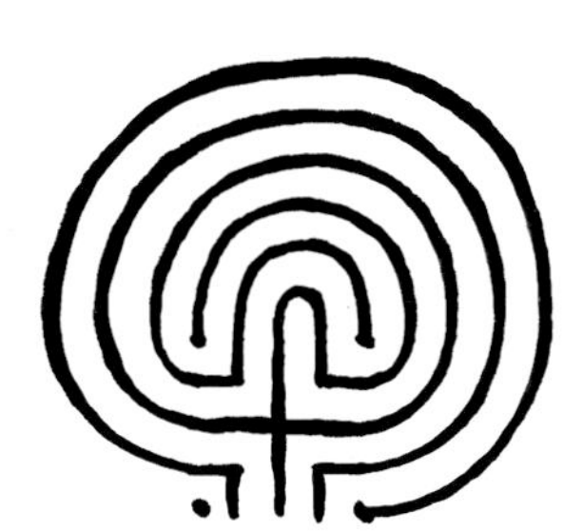

7 From the horizontal line of the bottom left-hand corner angle draw a wide arc to the bottom right-hand dot.

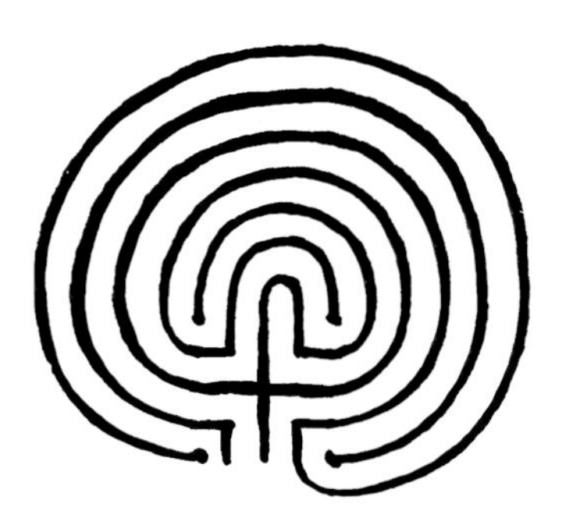

8 Connect the bottom left-hand dot with the vertical line of the bottom right-hand corner angle.

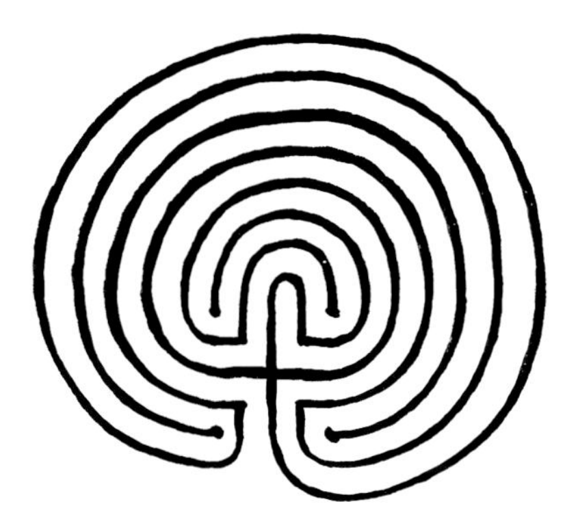

9 Finally, connect the vertical line of the bottom left-hand corner angle all the way over the top to the bottom of the vertical axis.

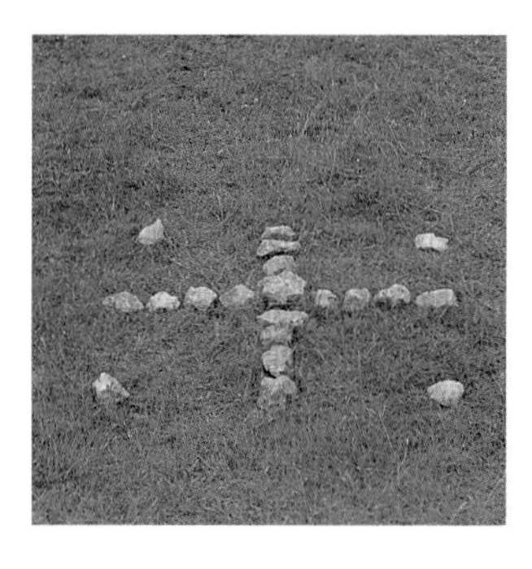

1 To make a three-circuit classical labyrinth arrange a number of stones in a cross and place a single stone in each quadrant. Allow a minimum of 1ft (30cm) between the center of your cross and each corner stone as this will define the width of the path.

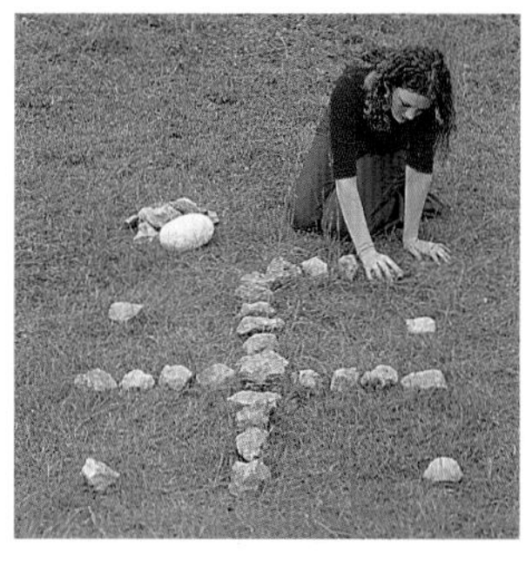

2 Make the crook shape first by connecting the top of the cross with the top right-hand corner stone. This will make a left-entry labyrinth. (To make a right-entry labyrinth connect the top of the cross with the top left-hand corner stone and exchange left for right in steps 3–5.)

Playing with the classical design

When you are familiar with the three- and seven-path classical designs experiment with different materials to make labyrinths of any size. If you have limited space available you could mold one with clay, carve one into wood, or simply paint one on to canvas. Let your brush choose the colors on your pallet!

If you would like to create a classical labyrinth that is large enough to walk, begin by marking one out with stones. Stone labyrinths are simple to make and easy to dismantle if you decide to assemble one in a public area. Ensure that you have a good supply of stones at hand, which you may find lying around naturally at your chosen site. Remember, removing stones permanently from beaches, in particular, can affect land erosion, so always replace them afterwards.

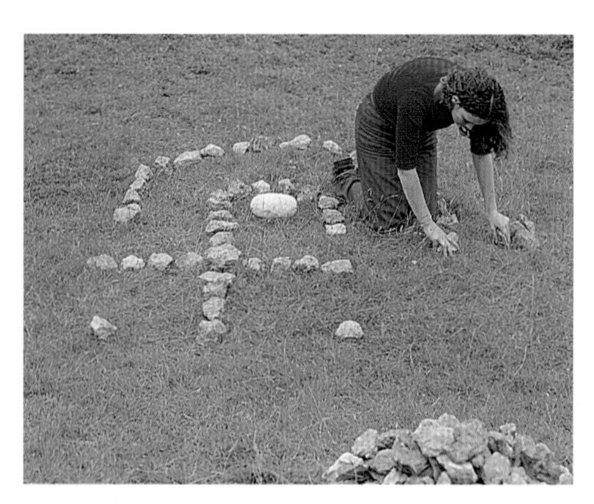

3 Return to the top left-hand corner stone and arrange an arc of stones to join up with the right horizontal line of the cross.

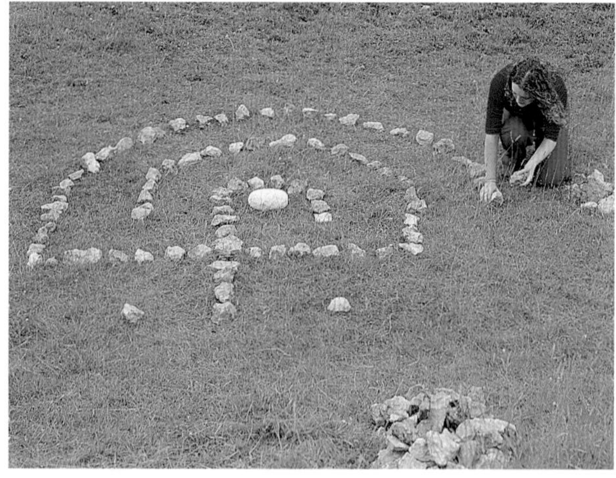

4 Now connect the left horizontal line of the cross with the lower right-hand corner stone.

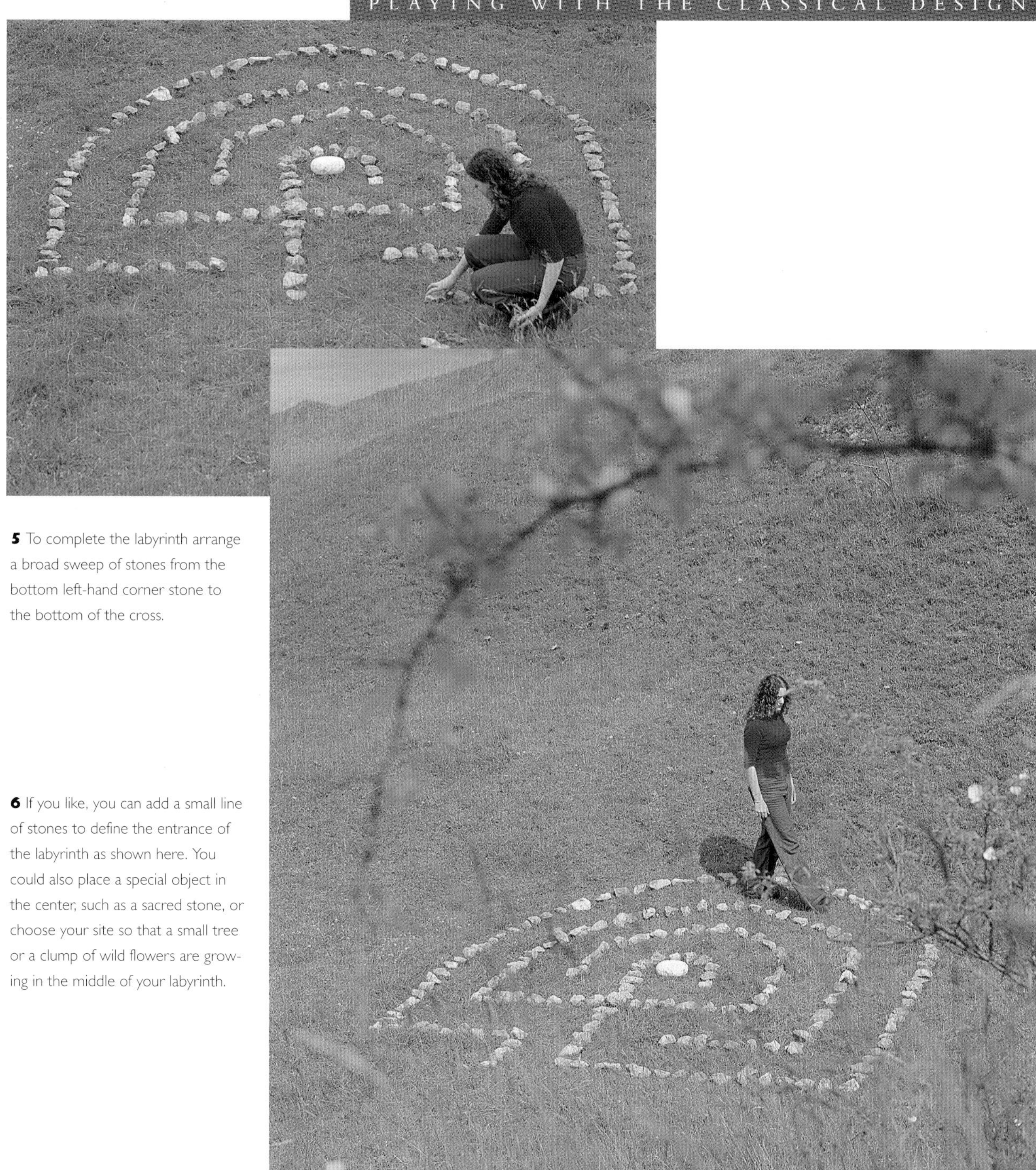

5 To complete the labyrinth arrange a broad sweep of stones from the bottom left-hand corner stone to the bottom of the cross.

6 If you like, you can add a small line of stones to define the entrance of the labyrinth as shown here. You could also place a special object in the center, such as a sacred stone, or choose your site so that a small tree or a clump of wild flowers are growing in the middle of your labyrinth.

Choosing different materials

Use your imagination when choosing materials to make labyrinths. This festive classical labyrinth in Plano, Illinois (below) was marked out with Christmas fairy lights on grass. You could make a similar labyrinth with string in your own garden. Follow the instructions on pp. 90–91, only this time mark the paths with brightly colored twine. You can fix it into the grass with U-pins or bits of bent wire.

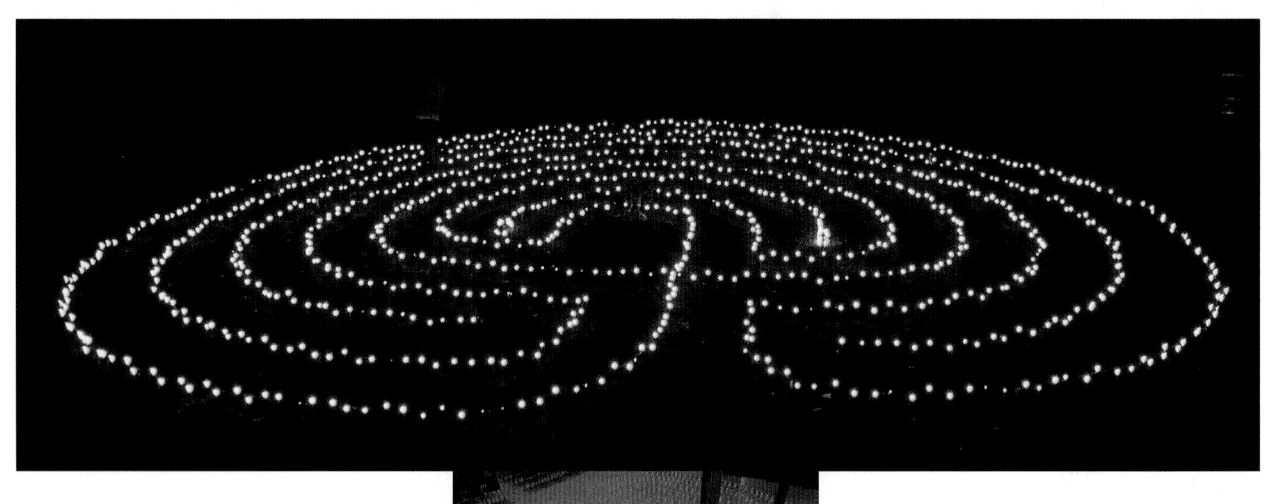

Lit candles in jam jars are another simple alternative to fairy lights, while hay bales will provide solid and sweet-smelling walls to walk in between. Another simple idea is to use masking tape on flooring or carpet.

The labyrinth (right) was made with surplus paper cups from the 2000 labyrinth festival at Saffron Walden in Essex, England.

Try thinking of other ideas that will recycle materials. The labyrinth on the facing page (near right) was made with scraps from commercial pallets in Kristianstad, Sweden, while the stones used for the design in Valbypark, Copenhagen (facing page, far right), were dredged from the River Øresund when building the bridge from Copenhagen in Denmark to Malmö in Sweden.

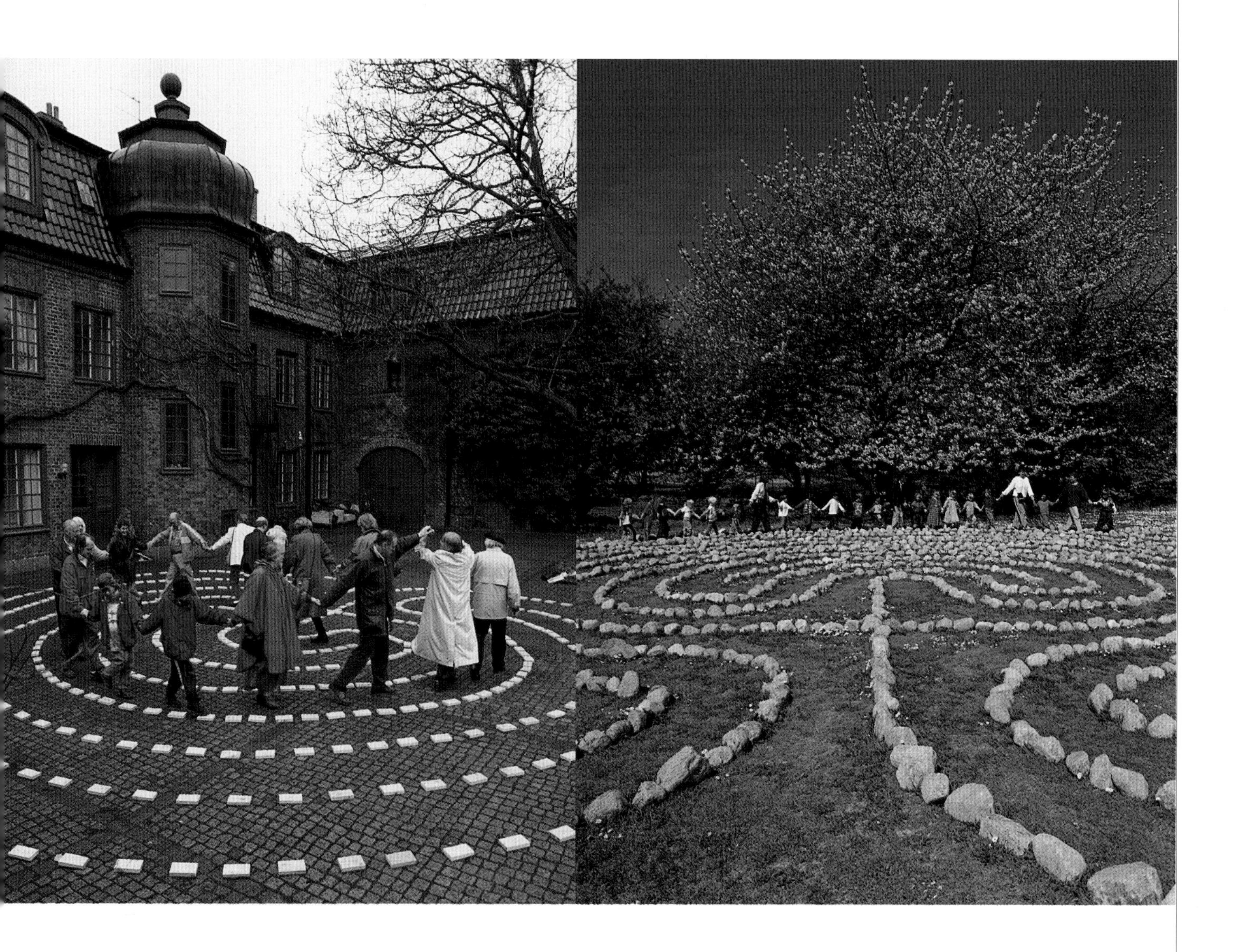

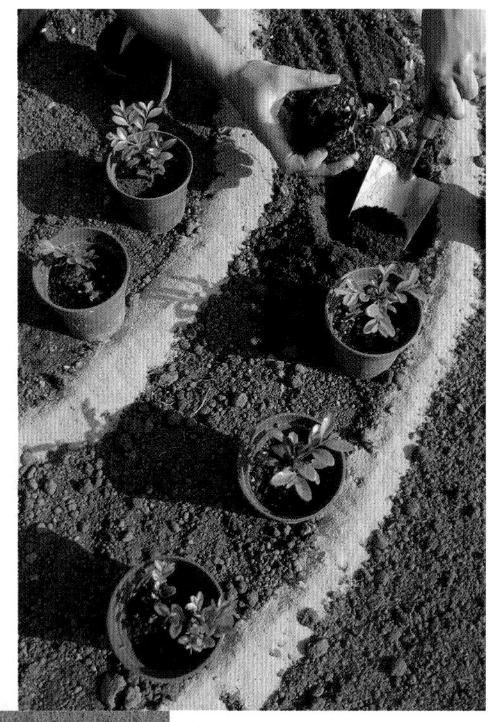

Other ideas for your garden

The labyrinth below was mown into the grass of a back garden and is great for dashing in and out of on summer afternoons. If your grass is not long enough, try drizzling circuits of sand on to your lawn to mark out the paths. You can then dampen the sand with a garden sprinkler to stop it from blowing away in the wind.

If you want something a little more permanent, you can plant a box hedge labyrinth (right) or fill a flowerbed with brightly colored bedding plants. A spring bulb labyrinth will welcome the new year.

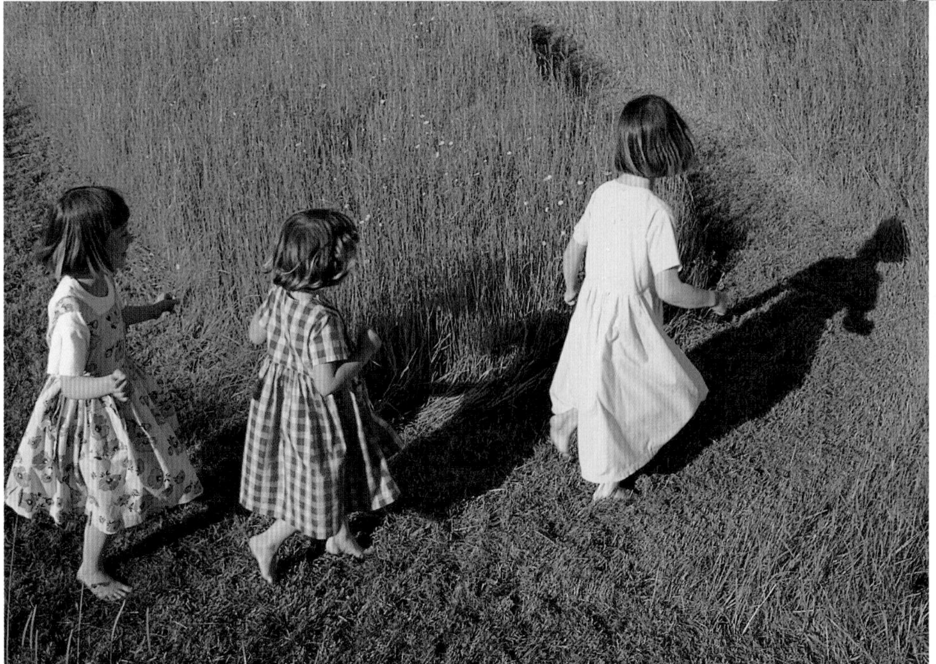

Labyrinths do not have to be big to enjoy. This labyrinth (right) was built into a garden patio.

To make your own, remove a paving slab from your patio and make sure the area underneath it is flat. Lay out your design in the space to check that you have the correct number of pebbles or shells. Remove these and pour dry-fix cement powder up to the level of the other patio stones. Arrange your design into the cement. To fix cement, wet the area with fine spray from a watering can.

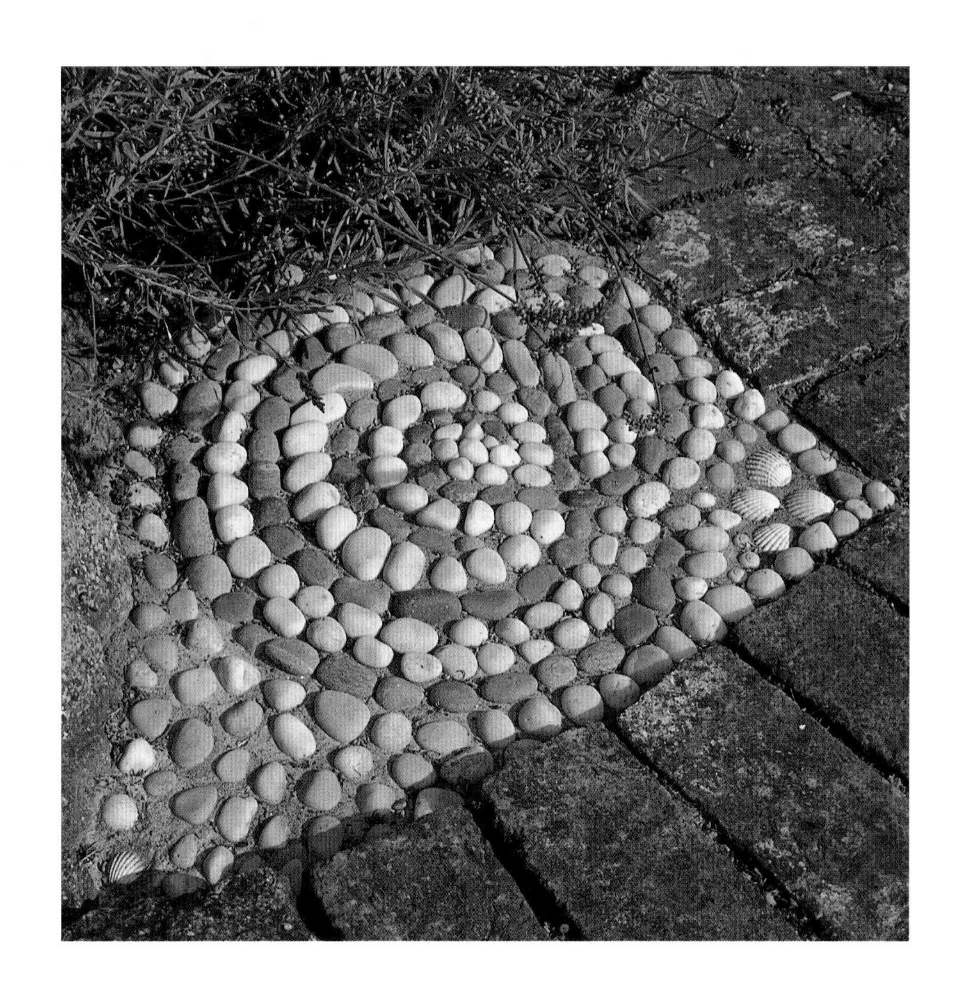

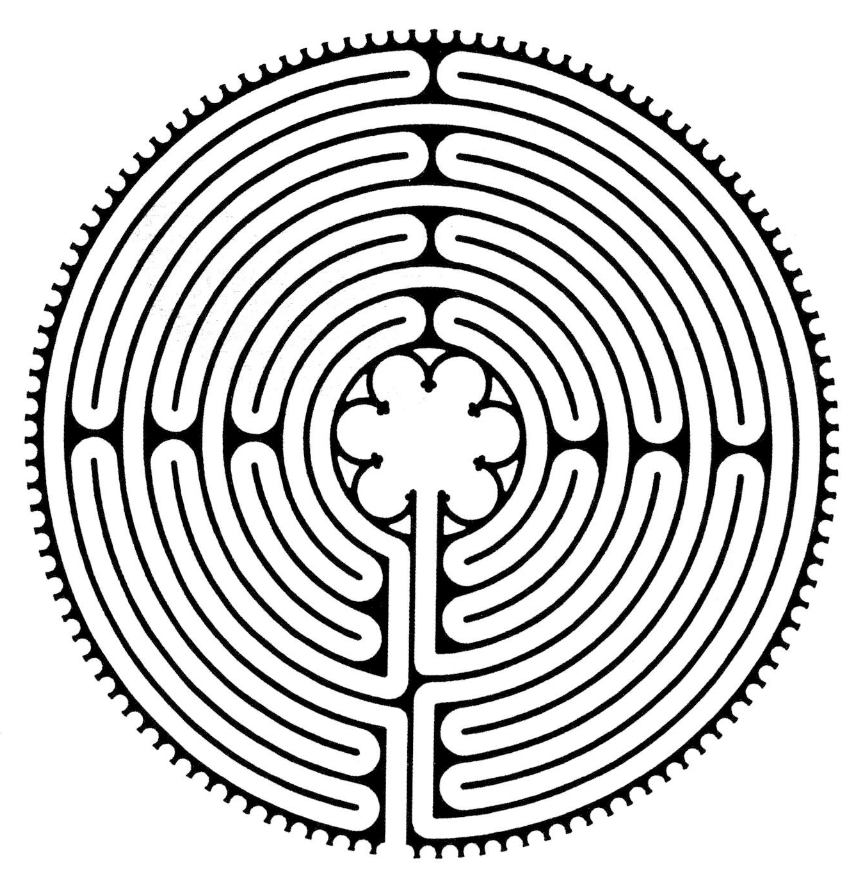

Studying the Chartres design

The Chartres labyrinth is an intricate design, measuring approximately 42.3 ft (12.9 m) across the east–west diameter, including lunations. Its grey-tone pathway is 861.5 ft (262.6 m) long and 13.4 inches (34 cm) wide, with 3.1 inch- (8 cm-) wide walls made from blue-black marble. It was built into the floor of the cathedral around 1194–1220, and lies in the aisle beneath the west rose window. It has 11 concentric circuits and a rose-petaled center measuring 9 ft (2.74 m) wide. The rose has six petals and is thought to symbolize the feminine, in particular Mary, Mother of Christ. The rose is also a symbol of spiritual enlightenment.

As you tread the pathway to the rose center, you explore the entire area of the labyrinth rather than each quadrant in turn. There are a total of 34 turns as you journey in. Twenty-eight of these are full U-turns and the remaining six are right-angle turns. If you look closely at the U-turns, you will see that 20 of them are separated by 10 labrys shapes (see p. 64).

Around the circumference of the labyrinth are teeth-like extensions called lunations.These consist of 112 cups and 113 cusps. The entrance/exit pathway is the equivalent of two cups and one cusp wide. These are unique to the Chartres design and thought to have helped follow lunar cycles (the 112 cups represent four 28-day lunar months). You don't have to reproduce these if you are making a temporary Chartres labyrinth, although they will add to the beauty and resonance of a permanent and accurate copy.

Top axis: there are a total of four labrys shapes, each separated by an open pathway. Each labrys shape is bracketed by two paths that double back on themselves to create a turn on the labyrinth path.

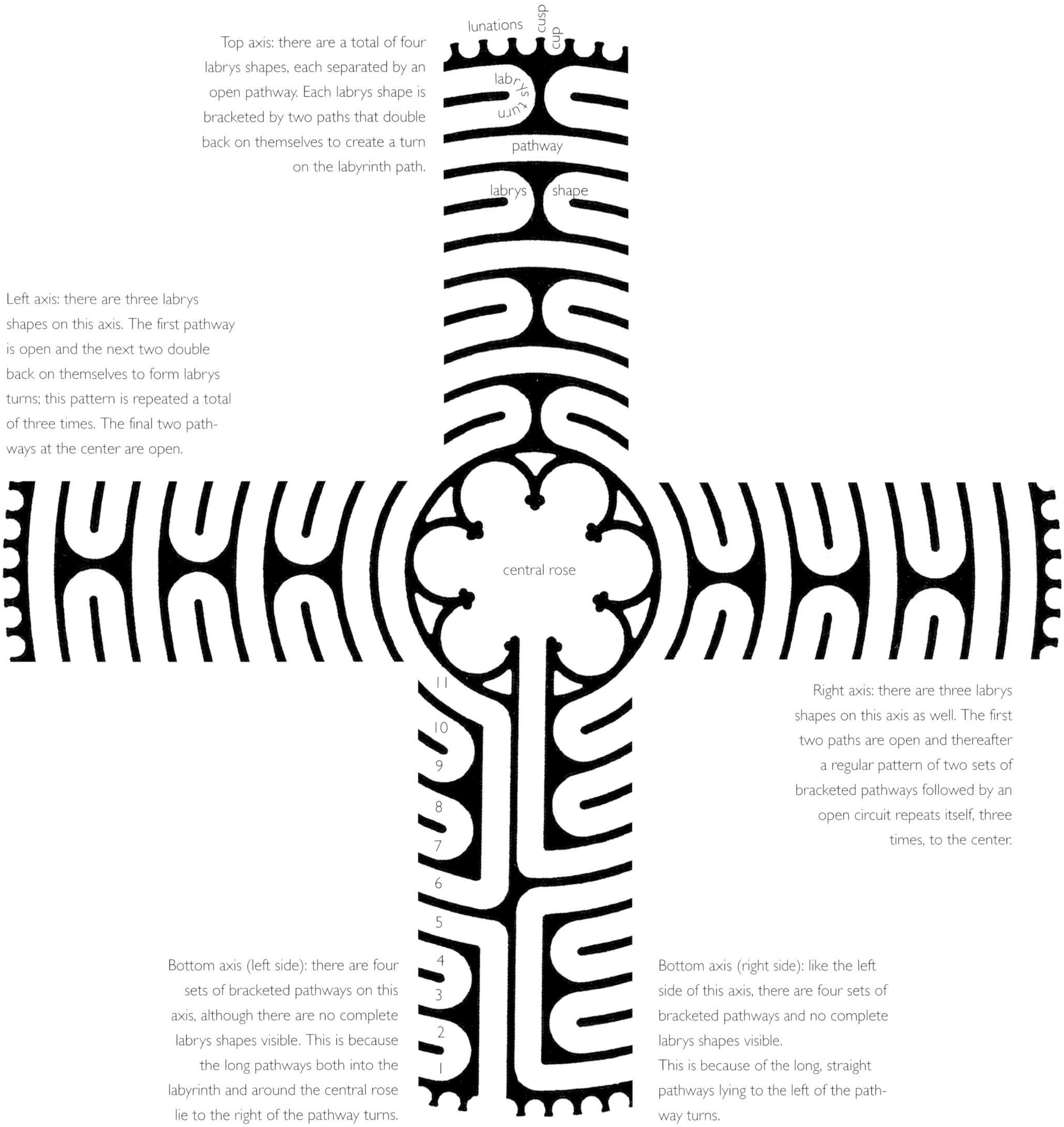

Left axis: there are three labrys shapes on this axis. The first pathway is open and the next two double back on themselves to form labrys turns; this pattern is repeated a total of three times. The final two pathways at the center are open.

Right axis: there are three labrys shapes on this axis as well. The first two paths are open and thereafter a regular pattern of two sets of bracketed pathways followed by an open circuit repeats itself, three times, to the center.

Bottom axis (left side): there are four sets of bracketed pathways on this axis, although there are no complete labrys shapes visible. This is because the long pathways both into the labyrinth and around the central rose lie to the right of the pathway turns.

Bottom axis (right side): like the left side of this axis, there are four sets of bracketed pathways and no complete labrys shapes visible.
This is because of the long, straight pathways lying to the left of the pathway turns.

Easy methods on sand or asphalt

Find a beach with a large expanse of untouched firm sand that is not too near the incoming tide. You will need at least one other person to help you make the labyrinth, as well as a long, thin rope or string and two strong sticks or lengths of wood cut from a broom handle. You will also need a picture of the Chartres design and a measuring stick cut to the intended width of the pathways (this should be at least 1 ft [30 cm] wide). If you feel confident without the rope and lengths of wood, you can just use your eye to calculate the circuits. The result will be a crude but exciting labyrinth to tread. Make sure you leave enough time to tread the labyrinth before the tide comes in!

If you decide to trace out the pathways with chalk on a large asphalt surface, such as a playground, you will need to tie the chalk on to the rope, draw a circuit and then unravel approximately 1 ft (30 cm) of rope to draw the next. Chalk in the labrys shapes and then rub out the pathway lines with your foot or a wet cloth to make the turns.

Making the circuits

1 Ask the person helping you to stand at the center of the space and to hold the stick with rope attached. Plant the stick in the sand, but keep hold of it so it remains upright and can swivel freely. This will be the center point of the labyrinth.

2 Decide how wide you want the labyrinth to be by tying one end of the rope on to the stick at the center, and the other on to the second stick. The distance between the two sticks will equal the radius of the entire labyrinth. Wind in the rope on your second stick until you are 3 ft (1 m) from the center point.

3 Walk around the person holding the stick and cut the circumference of the rose space into the sand.

4 Once you have traced the center space for the rose into the sand, let out about 1 ft (30 cm) of the rope and cut the first pathway in a full circle around the central circuit. Use the measuring stick to check that the path is wide enough.

5 Now unravel another 1 ft (30 cm) of rope to draw the second pathway, and repeat this until you have traced 12 continuous circuits (this includes the line marking the circumference of the rose space) into the sand.

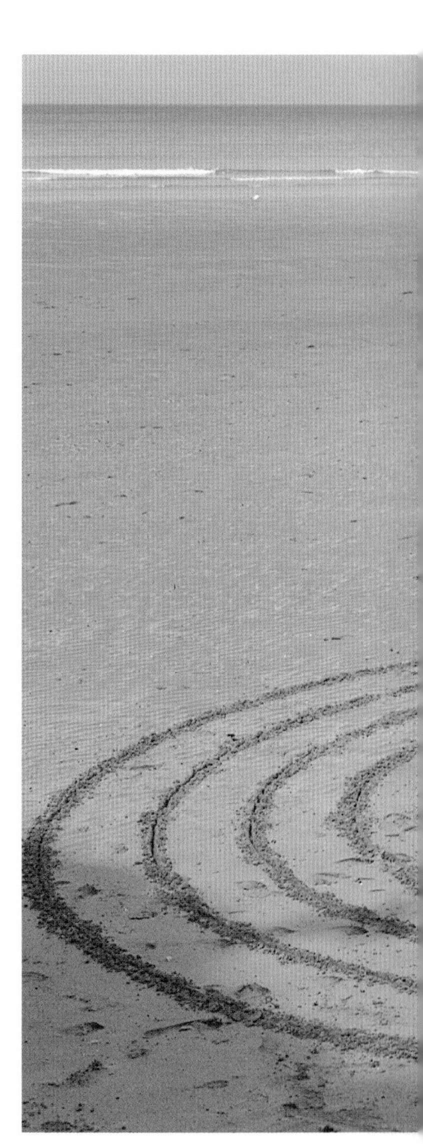

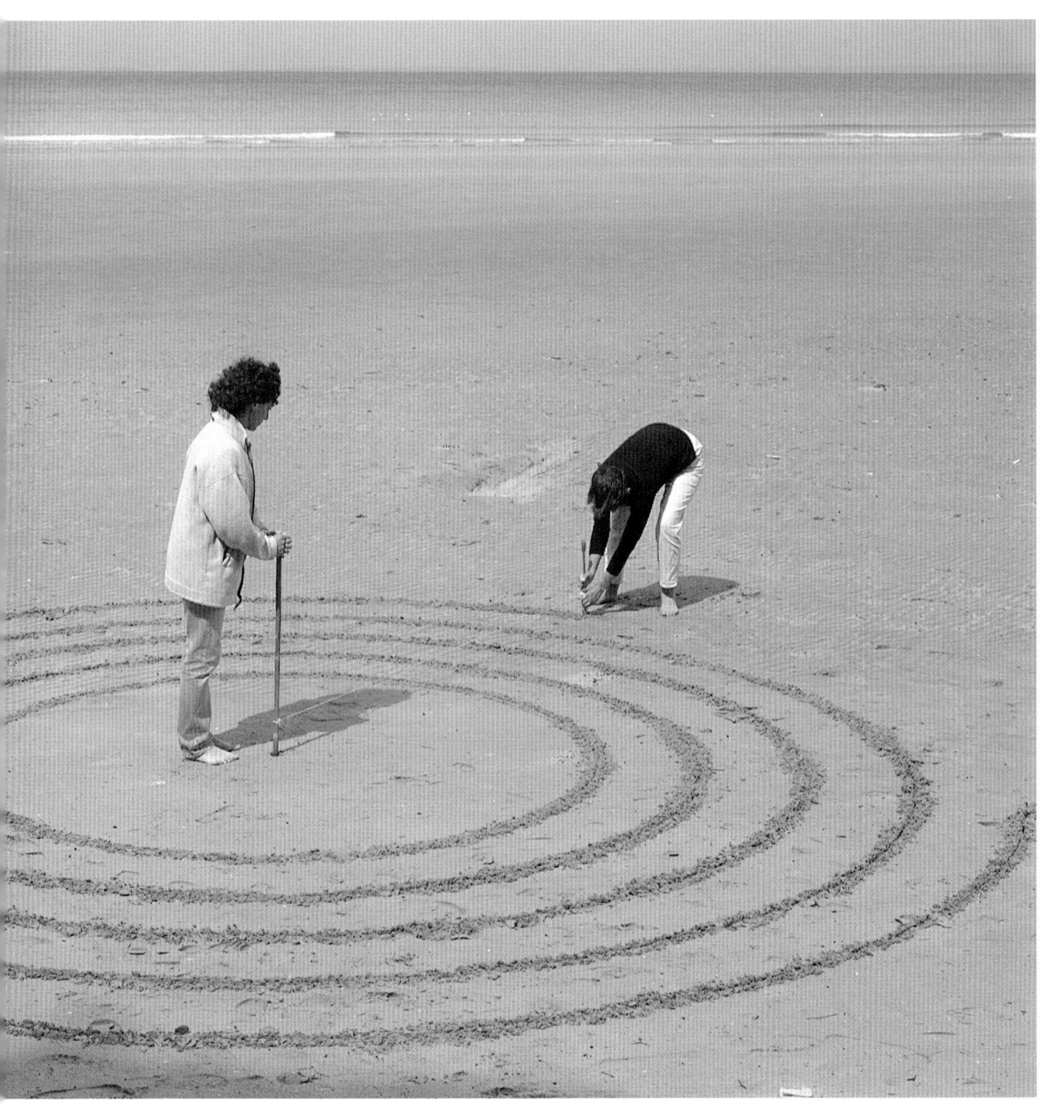

Making the labrys turns

Decide where you want the entrance/exit to lie (see Chapter Two to help you position your labyrinth). Mark the entrance, or bottom axis, on the circumference, as well as the top, left and right axes. Now consult the Chartres design on p. 97 to see which paths need to be made into labrys turns. Walk along each of the axes in turn, drawing in the labrys shapes and rubbing out the adjoining pathways to make the turns. There will be four labrys shapes in the top axis and three in the left and right. The bottom axis is a little more tricky.

1 Walk out in a straight line from the center of the labyrinth towards the bottom axis, rubbing out a 2 ft (60 cm) width as you go.

2 Divide this wide pathway into two with a single line from the circumference of the rose center to the outer circumference (call this the "stalk").

3 Look at the picture on p. 97. The left-hand pathway needs to join the fifth, sixth, and eleventh circuits. Rub out the lines to connect these circuits to the left stalk and draw in the four remaining labrys turns.

4 Now turn your attention to the right-hand path of the stalk. Rub out the sand so that it joins the first, sixth, and seventh circuits. Draw in the four remaining labrys turns. If you have time, add the six petals of the rose.

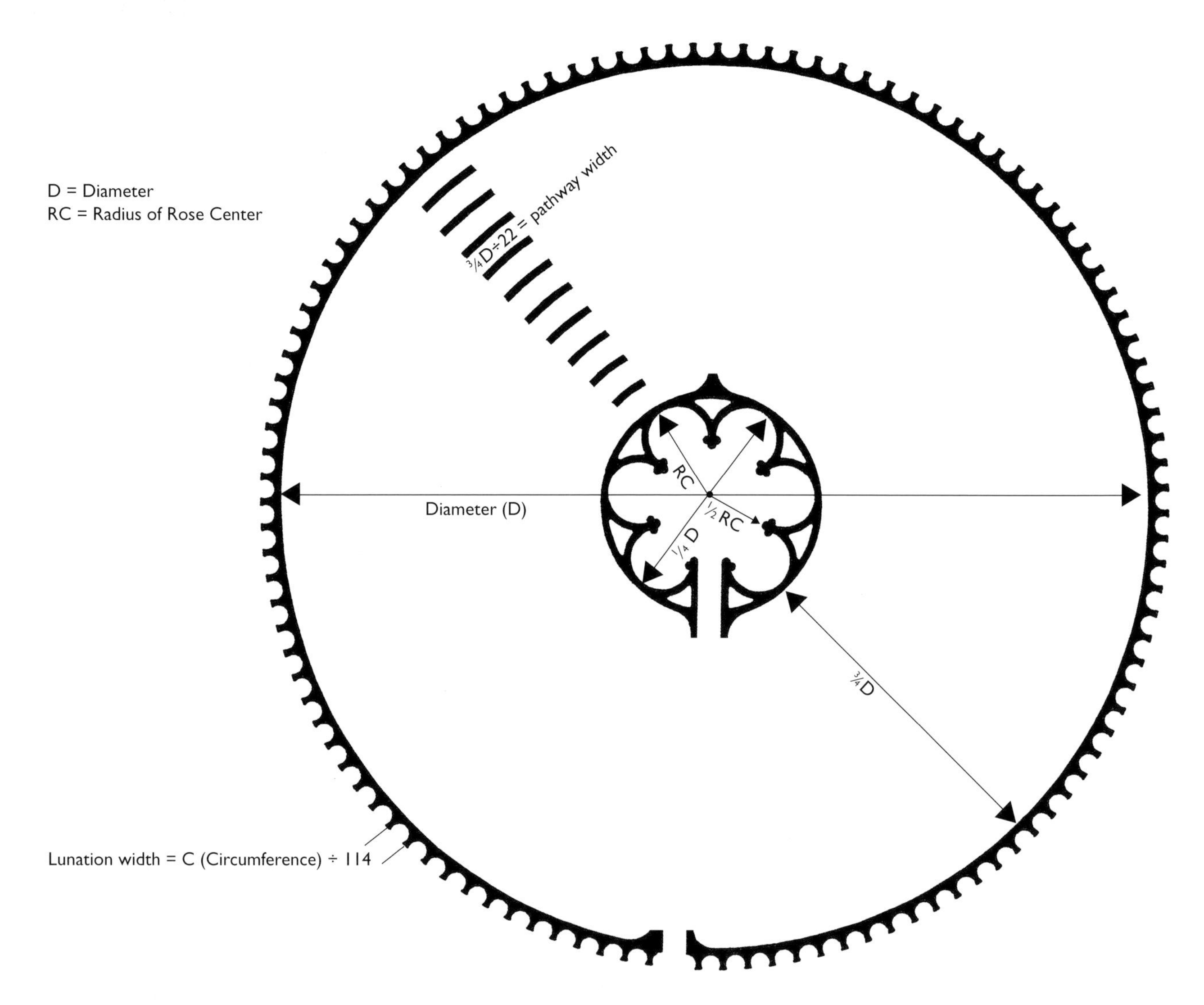

Precise method on canvas

Before you embark on a precise version of the Chartres labyrinth, you need to consider carefully where and how you intend to use your labyrinth. Will it be portable or do you intend to have it installed permanently in your garden? How durable should it be? Will it be walked by a handful of people or by several hundred? How will you transport it? A canvas labyrinth is very heavy and a luggage cart is often the answer. If you want to use it in public places, you may have to fireproof the material. Your budget may also affect the project.

Choose the material for your labyrinth on the basis of these considerations. The following pages focus on how to transfer the Chartres design on to canvas, although you can use the same formulas to calculate the precise dimensions for any Chartres project, large or small.

Calculating the dimensions

The dimensions of your labyrinth are usually dictated by two factors, namely the space you have available and the width of the pathways. The measurements of the labyrinth can be broken down into the following formulas, where:

D is the diameter of the labyrinth (excluding the height of the lunations);

RC is the radius of the rose center at the middle of the labyrinth. RC = ⅛ D;

C is the circumference of the labyrinth (excluding lunations). C = D × π (π is approx. 3.1416).

On the basis of D and RC we can calculate that:
• the diameter of the rose center = ¼ D;
• the width of the pathways = ¾ D ÷ 22 (there are 22 pathways), though note that this width also includes the lines separating the pathways.
• the distance from the indentations of the petals to the center of the labyrinth = ½ RC;
• the width of each lunation = C ÷ 114 (there are 112 lunation cups, plus the two that are absent from the entrance/exit of the labyrinth);
• the height of each lunation is approximately ⅔ of a pathway width.

Calculating from pathway width

If you want the pathway width to be 12 in (30 cm) you can calculate the dimensions of your labyrinth with the formula *pathway width = ¾ D ÷ 22.*

12 in (30 cm) x 22 = ¾ D
22 ft (6.6 m) = ¾ D
D = 22 ft (6.6 m) x 1 ⅓
D = 29.3 ft (8.8 m)

From this we can calculate the remaining dimensions of the labyrinth:

• *the diameter of the rose center is ¼ D*, i.e. 7.3 ft (2.2 m);
• *RC = ⅛ D*, or 3.7 ft (1.1 m);
• the distance from the indentations of the petals to the center of the labyrinth = *½ RC*, i.e. 22 in (55 cm);
• C = D x π, that is 90.6 ft (27.6 m);
• *the width of each lunation = C ÷ 114*, namely 9.5 in (24.3 cm);
• *the height of each lunation = ⅔ pathway width*, that is 8 in (20 cm);
• the height of lunations will increase the full diameter of the labyrinth by 16 in (40 cm), so the total diameter of the labyrinth is 30.6 ft (9.2 m).

Calculating from space available

No matter what space you have available, make sure you leave some room around the edge. For example, if you have 40 ft (12 m) available, make your working diameter about 36 ft (11 m).

When you have decided on the diameter of your design you can calculate the remaining dimensions using the formula where:

• *the width of the pathways = ¾ D ÷ 22*, that is 14.8 in (37.5 cm);
• *the diameter of the rose center = ¼ of D*, i.e. 9 ft (2.75 m);
• *RC = ⅛ D*, namely 4.5 ft (1.4 m);
• the distance from the indentations of the petals to the center of the labyrinth = *½ RC*, or 2.25 ft (69 cm);
• *the width of each lunation = C ÷ 114*, that is 11.9 in (30.3 cm);
• *the height of each lunation = ⅔ pathway width*, or 9.8 in (25 cm);
• the height of lunations will increase the diameter of the entire labyrinth by 19.6 in (50 cm), so the total diameter of the labyrinth will be 37.6 ft (11.3 m).

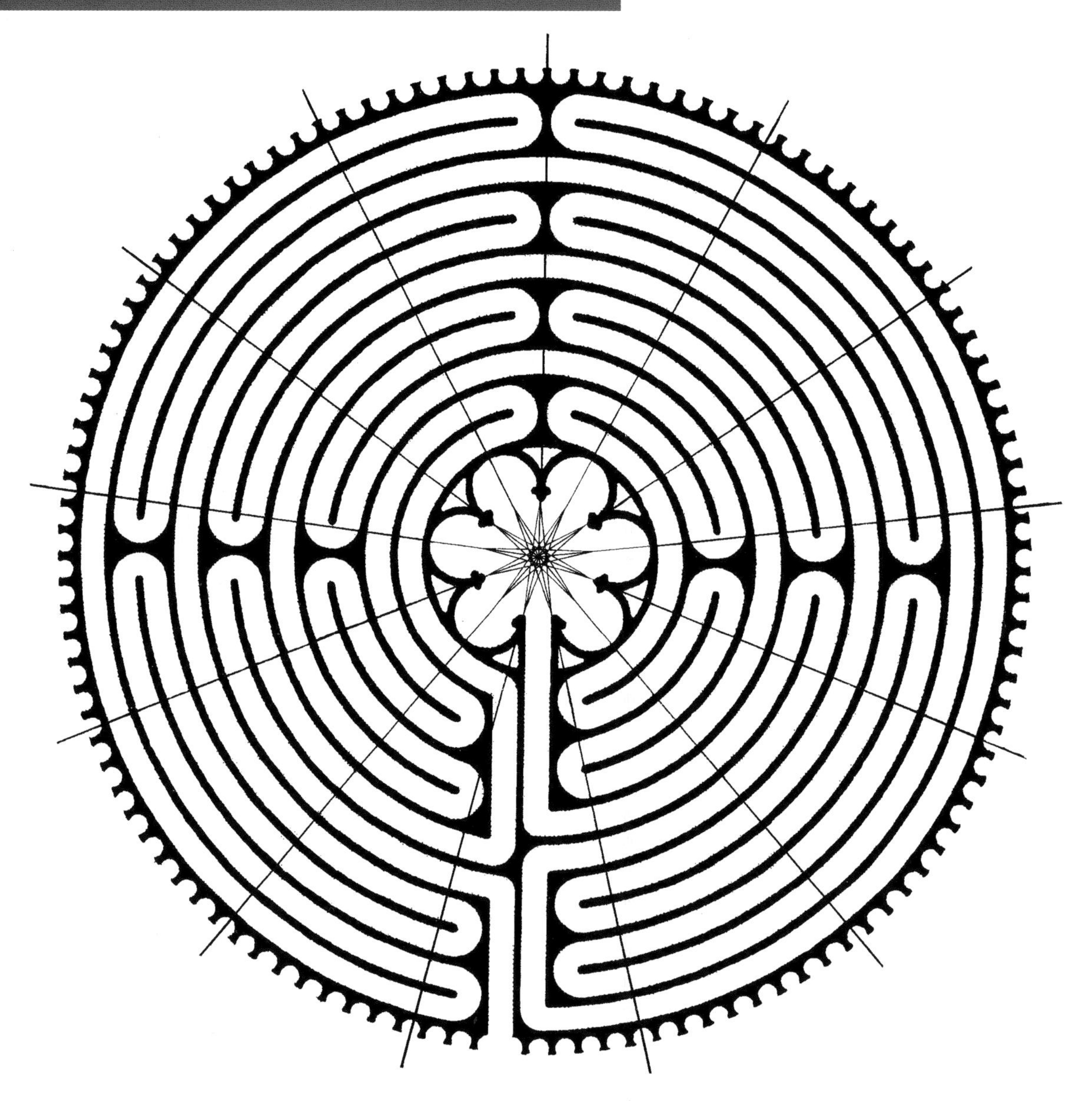

From design to material

When you have purchased and prepared the material you intend to use, such as canvas, and have calculated the dimensions for your labyrinth using the formula on p. 101, you can start to draw the design to scale on to your material base. Ask at least one other person to help you.

Before you begin, to keep this method as simple as possible, make stencils for the rose center, the entrance/exit path to the labyrinth, a lunation and a labrys shape (see right and p. 104). You will need large sheets of stiff paper, a length of firm, nonexpanding string, and a pencil. Once you have made the stencils you can start to pencil the design on to your material.

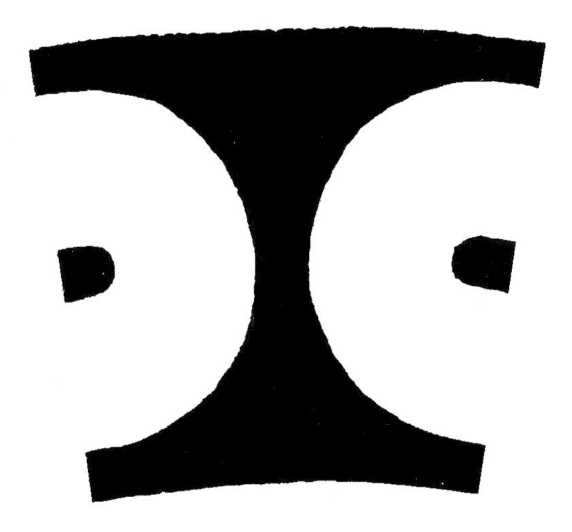

Rose center stencil

Before you start, you will need to photocopy the picture of the 13-point star superimposed over the labyrinth (left). This will help you position the petals of the rose and the entrance/exit path to the rose center.

1 Using a pencil attached to string rotating around the center point, draw the rose center circumference on to stiff paper. The diameter of the rose center is ¼ D (see p. 101).

2 Lay the photocopy of the labyrinth with the 13-point star on the stencil paper, centering it exactly on the stencil center. Fix it with sticky tape.

3 Look at the photocopy carefully. Notice how there are 13 lines extending from the points of the little 13-point star in the center of the labyrinth (see left).

Take a long ruler and lay it along one of these lines. Draw along it and out on to the stiff card, extending the line until you reach the outer diameter of the rose center. Draw out along each of the lines in turn until you have extended all 13 to the outer diameter of the rose center.

4 Look again at the photocopy. Each of the 13 lines either bisects one of the rose petals or crosses it at either side. Label these on the card. Notice how the entrance/exit path to the rose center is aligned with two of the lines. Label these as well.

5 Next mark where the six petals indent the inner circumference of the rose. Use the formula *petal indentation = ½ RC* (see p. 101) to calculate where this should be. The seven indentations will lie on seven of the lines you have drawn.

6 Using the 13 lines you transferred from the star to guide you, draw the petal arcs on to the card. (The center of each circle you draw to make the arcs is about a ¼ RC distance from the center of the labyrinth.) Note how the petal indentations end in little rounded crosses (see left). Cut around the petal shapes to make them easier to trace on to the canvas. There will be a gap between the first and sixth petals for the entrance/exit path to the rose center.

Entrance/exit pathway stencil

You can now make a long strip of paper two pathway-widths wide for the entrance/exit pathway (the width of the pathway is ¾ D ÷ 22, and the length of the entrance/exit pathway ½ D). Divide the stencil into two down the length of the card to make two pathways. The left pathway will be the entrance/exit path to the labyrinth, the right the path to the rose center.

Stencil for labrys shape

If you study the labrys shapes that separate the turns on the labyrinth you will see that they comprise two arcs lying back-to-back. The width of each labrys shape, or the diameter of each arc, is approximately twice that of the width you have chosen for the pathways (*pathway width = ¾ D ÷ 22*). Working from this measurement, draw two arcs back-to-back on a piece of card, leaving a small gap in between. Join the two arcs to make a labrys shape and cut out this shape for later.

Note: The two lines you draw to join the two arcs will probably be straight. However, if you study the Chartres design you will see that these actually curve with the labyrinth circuits. Do not worry as you only need this stencil for the shape of the arcs.

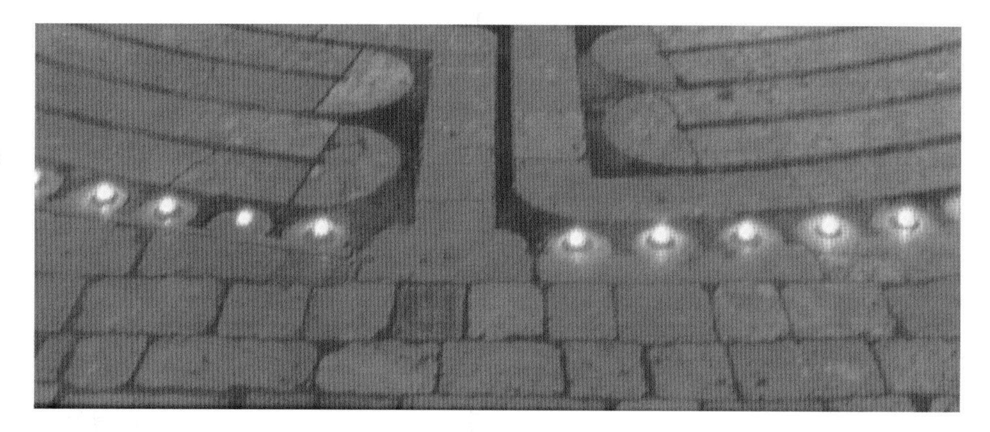

Stencil for lunations

Although it is best to mark the width of each lunation around the circumference of the labyrinth, a lunation stencil will make them easier to draw.

Lunations are made up of a curved cup-shape, within two containing lines or cusps. Note how the cusps are part of the arc forming the cup, and so are not straight-edged, but curve in slightly at the top.

1 Use the formula C ÷ 114 to find the lunation width.

2 Allowing for the thickness of the cusp line, draw two adjoining arcs on to a piece of card within the lunation width. (They should be ⅔ of a pathway width high.) Leave quite a fat base line and draw in the cusps on either side. Cut out for later.

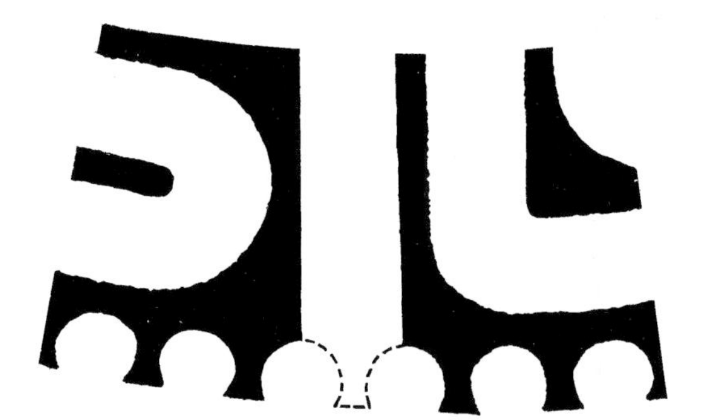

The entrance/exit to the labyrinth is the equivalent of two cups and one cusp wide. Remember to take these into account when calculating the position of the visible lunations around the circumference of the labyrinth.

Starting at the center

When you have made your stencils you can draw the labyrinth design on to canvas or other choice of material.

1 Find the center of the canvas with a measuring tape and mark it. Cut a hole in the center of your rose center stencil and place this over the center point of the canvas. Secure the stencil with sticky tape and draw around the rose petals. Remove the stencil.

2 Next align the entrance/exit stencil with the rose center that you have drawn on to the canvas. Tape this securely to the canvas and draw around it. Remove this stencil too.

You have now drawn the rose center as well as the entrance/exit pathways to the rose center and to the actual labyrinth.

Painting the labyrinth design

Once you have transferred the Chartres design on to the canvas, you can then begin to paint over the pencil marks. The paint you buy will be influenced by how you intend to use your canvas labyrinth: first, if the canvas is to be folded, then the paint has to be flexible and not crack; second, if the labyrinth is to be used outside, then the paint should also be waterproof. I used acrylic paint, thinned with PVA glue, which gave it a flexible, water-resistant finish. Make sure you allow the paint to dry thoroughly before you attempt to fold up the canvas. If you are going to use the canvas outside, you should also consider buying large plastic sheeting from a hardware supplier. This will prevent the canvas from getting wet from condensation on the ground.

Creating a Chartres labyrinth in this way is a time-consmuing but extremely rewarding project, which you and others can enjoy for many years. This method is intended to help you make an accurate copy of the Chartres design in the simplest possible way. However, if you find your labyrinth is not wholly accurate, don't worry, as it should not affect your experience on its path. In the same way, whatever design of labyrinth you experiment with, be it large or small, indoors or outdoors, ultimately it is your journey on it that is important and the fun you have in the making.

Drawing the pathways

3 Ask the person helping you to hold a strong stick or spindle upright on the center point of the canvas. Their job is to ensure the spindle stays in place while allowing it to rotate smoothly.

4 Attach a long length of firm, non-expanding string to the bottom of the stick.

5 Using the dimensions you calculated on p. 101, mark RC (radius of the rose center) on to the cord, measuring from the stick and out along the string.

6 Twine the cord firmly around a thick pencil at this mark. Hold the cord taut and walk the pencil around the center to draw the first circle. Be careful to keep the pencil vertical and not to let it slope sideways, as this will distort the circle. This circuit should match up with the petals you drew with the rose center stencil.

7 Starting from the first mark you made on the cord, RC, now measure the first pathway width. Mark this point on the string and wind it around the pencil. Draw the pathway as before and continue in this way until you have drawn all 12 circuits (there are 12 including the circumference of the rose center).

Labrys turns and lunations

8 You now need to draw in the labrys shapes using the stencil you prepared on p. 103 and connect the pathways marked with the entrance/exit stencil to the rest of the labyrinth's circuits.

Consult the picture on p. 97 to see where the paths need to be bracketed to form labrys turns. There are four labrys shapes at the top of the design and three to the left and right. The entrance/exit pathways are a little more complicated: first, you will need to draw half labrys shapes by hand; second, you will need to join the entrance/exit pathways to the labyrinth circuits.

9 Finally, you can draw on the lunations. These are quite tricky as they are not evenly distributed on the original design. Working from the formula, *lunation width = C ÷ 114*, mark the 114 lunations around the circumference of the labyrinth.

When you are satisfied with your marks, use the stencil you prepared opposite as a rough guide to draw on the lunations. Notice how the cusps are offset at the entrance and that there is a cusp directly on the north axis. You will draw on a total of 113 cusps and 112 cups, leaving the equivalent of one cusp and two cups for the entrance/exit of the labyrinth.

Bibliography

Artress, L. *Walking a Sacred Path.* New York: Riverhead Books, 1995.

Attali, J. *The Labyrinth in Culture and Society: Pathways to wisdom.* Berkeley: North Atlantic Books, 1999.

Bord, J. *Mazes and Labyrinths of the World.* London: Latimer New Dimensions, 1976.

The Chalice Well and Gardens, Glastonbury (booklet). Chalice Well Trust. Glastonbury

Champion, A. *My Involvement in Labyrinths.* Essex: Labyrinthos, 2000.

Charitonidou, A. *Epidaurus: The sanctuary of Asclepios and the museum.* Athens: Clio Editions, 1978.

Charpentier, L. *The Mysteries of Chartres Cathedral.* Suffolk: RILKO Books, 1993.

The Concise Oxford Dictionary of English Literature. Oxford: Oxford University Press, 1957.

Cooper, J. C. *An Illustrated Encyclopedia of Traditional Symbols.* London: Thames & Hudson, 1992.

Critchlow, K., J. Carroll, & L.V. Lee. *Chartres Maze: A model of the universe?.* Cambridge: RILKO Trust, 1975.

Fisher, A., & G. Gerster. *The Art of the Maze.* London: Weidenfeld & Nicolson, 1990.

Fisher, A., & D. Kingham. *Mazes.* Princes Risborough: Shire Pubns, 1991.

Graves, R. *The Greek Myths.* St. Ives: Penguin Books, 1992.

Houvet, E. *An Illustrated Monograph of Chartres Cathedral.* Chartres: Houvet, E., 1928.

Jaskolski, H. *The Labyrinth: Symbol of fear, rebirth and liberation.* Boston & London: Shambhala, 1997.

Kern, H. *Through the Labyrinth.* Munich, London & New York: Prestel, 2000.

Kraft, J. *The Goddess in the Labyrinth.* Finland: Abo Akademi, 1995.

Kroll, U. *In Touch with Healing.* London: BBC Books. 1991.

Lonegren, S. *Labyrinths: Ancient myths and modern uses.* Glastonbury: Gothic Image Pubns., 1996.

Martineau, J. *Mazes and Labyrinths in Great Britain.* Wales: Wooden Books, 1996.

Matthews, W. H. *Mazes and Labyrinths: Their history and development.* New York: Dover. 1970.

Michell, J. *The New View over Atlantis.* London: Thames & Hudson, 1995.

Miller, H., & P. Broadhurst. *The Sun and the Serpent.* Cornwall: Pendragon Press, 1994.

Miller, M. *Chartres Cathedral.* Andover: Pitkin, 1995.

Miller, M. *Chartres Cathedral: Stained glass and sculpture.* Andover: Pitkin Pictorials Ltd., 1990.

Purce, J. *The Mystic Spiral: Journey of the soul.* London: Thames & Hudson, 1977.

Saward, J. *Ancient Labyrinths of the World.* Essex: Caerdroia, 1999.

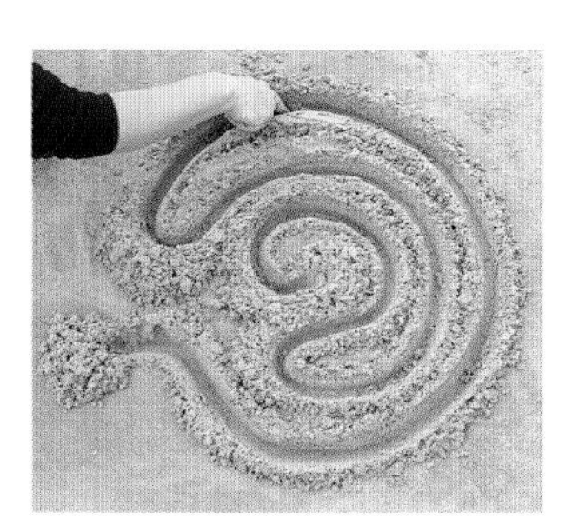

Saward, J. (ed.). *Caerdroia: The journal of mazes and labyrinths.* Essex: Caerdroia, 1999.

Waters, F. *Book of the Hopi.* Harmondsworth: Penguin Books, 1977.

White, R. *Working with your Chakras.* London: Piatkus, 1993.

Wosien, M. G., *Sacred Dance: Encounter with the gods.* New York: Thames & Hudson, 1986.

Gazetteer

The labyrinths detailed below are a selection of the most interesting and accessible examples in each given country. Consult web sites for comprehensive listings.

Australia & New Zealand

There are a handful of walkable, public labyrinths, including those at:

Crystal Castle near Mullumbimby, NSW, which has a new turf and stone Chartres design. For details email castle@spot.com.au or visit *www.crystalcastle.net*

The Brookfield Centre in Brisbane, Queensland (outdoor labyrinth). Email cmlander@medeserv.com.au

Frederic Wallis House in Lower Hutt, Wellington (outdoor labyrinth). Email fwallis@paradise.net.nz.

Consult web sites on p. 108 for details of other new labyrinths.

Austria

There are a many new labyrinths here, especially in parks and gardens. Notable examples include those at Salzburg, Innsbruck, Pöllau, Obdach, Bad Loipersdorf, Bad Tatzmansdorf, Kaltenbrunn, Heiligenkreuz and Südstadt Church, Vienna. Check web site on p. 109 for details.

Belgium

Ghent Town Hall. A rectangular pavement labyrinth measuring 39 × 46 ft. (12 × 14 m). Laid in 1528 and in excellent condition.

Canada

St. Paul's Anglican Church, Jervis Street, Vancouver, is home to a modern pavement labyrinth, a replica of the Chartres labyrinth.

Denmark

There are numerous 15th-century labyrinth frescoes in churches. The best are at Hesslager in southeast Fyn, Roerslev in northwest Fyn and Skive in northern Jylland.

Many recent stone labyrinth replicas are also worth visiting, such as those in the Lejre Centre, Sjælland (a 50 ft. [15 m] wide, 11-circuit, classical labyrinth), Valbypark in southwest Copenhagen (see p. 93) and at the Labyrinth Park in Rodelund, Jutland.

Finland

Home to many stone labyrinths. Those to survive are usually on remote offshore islands. The Åland archipelago, halfway between Finland and Sweden, has the best collection.

You can walk a modern *Jungfrudans* labyrinth (many Finnish labyrinths are called *Jungfrudans*, or maiden's dance) in the Bragegården on the edge of Vaasa, central Finland.

Worth seeing also are four 15th-century labyrinth frescoes in the church of St. Mary (Maaria Kyrka) on the outskirts of Turku.

France

Although some 20 examples of labyrinths are recorded in churches and cathedrals, some have been destroyed or are only architectural details. Several are in buildings with limited access. Three examples of walkable pavement labyrinths are recommended for visitors.

Chartres Cathedral: laid sometime between 1194 and 1220, this splendidly preserved example (see p. 18) is often covered with chairs. These are sometimes removed just before closing time to allow pilgrims to walk the labyrinth. Occasionally, it will still be uncovered when the cathedral reopens in the morning.

Amiens Cathedral: similar in design to the one at Chartres, but octagonal. The labyrinth is actually an 1894 replica of the original, which was constructed circa 1280, but destroyed in 1825. It too is often covered with chairs.

St. Quentin: this 1485 copy of the original Amiens labyrinth is in the Collegiate Church in the town center. It is in good condition and is usually uncovered and available for walking.

The 16th-century labyrinth in St Omer Cathedral is also worth visiting, although it is partly covered with candlesticks and kneelers. Laid in black and white marble, it is situated in front of the altar.

Germany

Three ancient turf labyrinths survive in Germany. The first is in a clearing in the Eilenriede forest, east of Hannover. It measures 105 ft. (32 m) in diameter and has a fully grown lime tree at its center.

Two smaller examples can be found near Leipzig, in the villages of Steigra and Graitschen. Consult the German web site for details of new labyrinths—there are several.

India

A number of stone labyrinths similar to those in Scandinavia survive in southern India, particularly in the state of Tamil Nadu (formerly Madras). Details of these are elusive.

There are also at least three stone reliefs in the Hoysaleshvara and Kedareshvara Temples in Halebid, Mysore.

Ireland

The oldest labyrinth in Ireland, dating to the early Christian period, is the Hollywood stone, decorated with a labyrinth measuring 28 in. (73 cm) wide. Discovered in County Wicklow, it is now kept in The National Museum of Ireland, Dublin.

Réált na Mara, Na Forbacha, County na Gaillimhe, is a new stone Chartres replica you can walk.

Italy

Two important examples are easily accessible: the small, 12th-century labyrinth carved into the north porch of Lucca Cathedral, measuring 20 in. (50 cm) wide; and the black and white, 16th-century marble labyrinth (11 ft. [3.4 m] in diameter) built into the floor of the San Vitale basilica, Ravenna.

Netherlands

Interesting examples include: St. Servaas Church, Maastricht, a 19th-century pavement labyrinth, similar to that in St. Omer, France, but often covered; Waalkade, Nijmegen, a stone pathway labyrinth bordered by channels filled with water; Kerkplein, Ruurlo, a decorative brick paving labyrinth; Wetenschap, Asenray, a modern stone labyrinth outside a former chapel, now an art gallery. See web site for further details.

Norway

A number of stone labyrinths are preserved in Norway, especially in the far north. Most are difficult to find without local guidance. Two 15th-century frescoes are preserved in the churches at Seljord and Vestre Slidre in the south.

Portugal

An impressive collection of four Roman mosaic labyrinths can still be seen among the ruins of Conimbriga in modern Coimbra.

South Africa

Pietermaritzburg Cathedral in Natal has a replica of the pavement labyrinth at Ely Cathedral, England. Installed in the porch in 1981.

Spain

There are a number of petroglyphs believed to date from around 900–500 B.C. on the hillsides above Pontevedra, Galicia, although these are difficult to find without local assistance. Also impressive is a Roman mosaic labyrinth preserved at Italica, near Seville.

Sweden

Some 300 or so stone labyrinths have been recorded in Sweden, but many of the surviving examples are in remote locations or on offshore islands. Two easily accessible examples are listed below.

Ulmekäar, northern Bohuslän: there is a beautifully preserved stone labyrinth, near the town of Grebbestad, an area famous for rock art and other prehistoric monuments.

Island of Gotland: Visby is probably the most famous stone labyrinth in Scandinavia (see p. 30), just north of the town of Visby. The island also has a number of other stone labyrinths and church frescoes.

Switzerland

Since 1991 some 60 labyrinths have been constructed in Switzerland, many in the grounds of churches and associated community and conference centers. Notable examples can be found in Baar, Basel, Bubikon, Lenzburg, Männedorf, Niedergösgen, St. Gallen, and Zürich.

Russia

A remarkable group of some 40 or so stone labyrinths still survives in the Solovetski Archipelago around the southern shore of the White Sea. Travel to this remote region is difficult.

United Kingdom

Eight historic turf labyrinths survive in England. The following are open to walk during daylight hours: Dalby, North Yorkshire; Alkborough, Lincolnshire; Wing, Rutland (see p. 53); Hilton, Cambridgeshire; Saffron Walden in Essex (see pp. 34–35); and St. Catherine's Hill, Winchester, in Hampshire (see p. 5). They range in size from 26 ft. (8 m) at Dalby to 131 ft. (40 m) at Saffron Walden.

A fascinating group of stone labyrinths can be found on the Scilly Islands. The original example (see p. 30) is on St. Agnes. Other later copies can be found on St. Mary's and especially on St. Martin's.

The only surviving medieval church labyrinth is a gilded roof boss in St. Mary's Redcliffe, Bristol.

The 19th-century labyrinth in Ely Cathedral is especially worth visiting, as is the collection of labyrinth details in Watts Chapel, Compton, Surrey.

There is also a canvas labyrinth project at the University of Dundee, Scotland, illustrated on pp. 58–59. See p. 109 for contact details.

United States of America

New labyrinths continue to appear throughout the U.S., so consult the web sites for the latest additions. Many are on private property, but the following are in public locations and well worth a visit.

Grace Cathedral, San Francisco: a replica of the Chartres labyrinth in woven carpet (see p. 57). This is the labyrinth that sparked the current revival of labyrinths in the U.S.

New Harmony, Indiana: a full-sized granite replica of the Chartres labyrinth, near the Historic New Harmony visitor center (see p. 38).

Naperville, Illinois: situated in Riverwalk Park, this beautiful replica of the Chartres labyrinth was made with hand-cut paving bricks.

Sibley Park, California: there are a number of recent stone labyrinths in this regional park between Oakland and Berkeley.

Tuscon, Arizona: a walkable pavement Pima labyrinth (see p. 37 for Pima design) is situated just off Speedway, outside a shopping mall.

West Palm Beach, Florida: a large turf labyrinth, built in 1997, outside the Norton Museum of Art.

Organizations/ magazines/ web sites

Australia

Jeff Trahair
The Adelaide Labyrinth Project
36 Thirkell Avenue
Beaumont 5066 SA
Tel: +61 (0)8 8379 7867
www.adelaide.net.au

Teia McCullough
Labyrinth Walkers Support Group
154 Mill Point Road, Unit 114
South Perth 6151 WA
Tel: +61 (0)8 9368 6294

UK

Labyrinthos & Caerdroia
(Journal of mazes and labyrinths)
Jeff Saward
53 Thundersley Grove
Thundersley, Benfleet
Essex SS7 3EB
Tel: +44 (0)1268 751915
jeff@labyrinthos.net
www.labyrinthos.net

University of Dundee
The Labyrinth Tapestry
The Chaplaincy Centre
Dundee DD1 4HN
Tel: +44 (0)1382 344157
n.r.halpin@dundee.ac.uk
www.insightsworld.com

For Information from Peter Dawkins on earth energy and Zoence Academy contact:
Sarah Dawkins
Roses Farmhouse
Epwell Road, Upper Tysoe
Warwick CV35 0TN
Tel: +44 (0)1295 688185
Fax: +44 (0)1295 680770
secretary@zoence.com
www.zoence.com

U.S.A.

Robert Ferré
128 Slocum Avenue
St. Louis, MO 63119
Tel: +1 314 968-5557
Fax: +1 314 968-5539
robert@labyrinthproject.com
www.labyrinthproject.com

The Labyrinth Society
PO Box 144
New Canaan, CT 06840-0144
Tel: +1 877 446-4520
labsociety@aol.com
www.labyrinthsociety.org

Veriditas
The Worldwide Labyrinth Project
Grace Cathedral
1100 California Street
San Francisco, CA 94108
Tel: +1 415 749-6358
veriditas@gracecathedral.org
www.gracecathedral.org

Europe

Consult the websites below for further information on European labyrinth locations:
Austria: *www.labyrinthe.at*
Germany: *www.begehbare-labyrinthe.de*
Netherlands:
www.smartbits.nl/labyrinth

Materials

When choosing material for my project I considered silk for its lightweight properties and cotton for ease of cleaning. However, I eventually decided on 12 oz. (340 g) natural cotton duck canvas. This would be durable and also not move too much when laid down. You can buy canvas from theatrical and artists' suppliers, who will also sew the lengths together. Remember to allow for some of the overall width of the material to be lost in seams and hems.

Theatrical and Artists' Suppliers (Canvas)
Russell and Chapple Ltd
23 Monmouth Street
Shaftesbury Avenue
London WC2H 9DE
UK
Tel: +44 (0)20 7836 7521

Artist Suppliers (Paint)
Atlantis European Ltd
146 Brick Lane
London E1 6RU
UK
Tel: +44 (0)20 7377 8855

Circle Dance

For comprehensive listings of international Circle Dance teachers

Grapevine
(Quarterly journal of the Sacred Circle Dance network)
Sally Maxwell
60 Bishop Road
Bristol BS7 8LT
Tel: +44 (0)117 9232115
sally@rotherfold.freeserve.uk

Circle Dance, Sacred Dance
(Quarterly Circle Dance newsletter)
John Bear
1107 Everglades
Pacifica, CA 94044
U.S.A.
john@ursa.net

Music

For recorded version of *Tsakonikos* and other Circle Dance music contact:
Frances Fawkes
Grapevine editor
4 Higher Brookfield Terrace
Lustleigh
Devon TQ13 9TW
UK
Tel: +44 (0)1647 277227
france.fawkes@lineone.net

Jennifer Berezan's *Returning*
Edge of Wonder Records
PO Box 6181
Albany, CA 94706
U.S.A.
Tel/Fax: +1 510 524-4183
berezan@sirius.com
www.edgeofwonder.com

Cantiones Sacrae (medieval music)
Barbara Swetina
Findhorn Foundation
The Park
Forres IV36 0TZ
UK
Tel/Fax: +44 (0)1309 690623

The Best of Márta Sebestyén
Hannibal, a Rykodisc label
Shetland Park
27 Congress Street
Salem, MA 01970
U.S.A.

Index

Acknowledgments

Author's acknowledgments

My thanks to

The makers and co-creators of the labyrinth canvas and journey: Geneviève Khemtemourian, Thierry Jacques, Sally Tombleson, June Hyde, Roberto del Pino, Sue & John Murray, Valerie Lesniak, Helen & Ray Armstrong, Marian Dunlea.

Those who encouraged and helped in countless ways: my daughters Rosie & Amy Sands, Jean Kirkpatrick, Robbie Ginsborg, Diana Wright, Julie & Freddy Dunstan, John Cassayd-Smith, David Standley, Zoe Fairbairns, Anaïs Simon, Sotos Alexandridis, Clive & Kerstin Lindley-Jones, Jeff Saward, Robert Gutsell, Croydon Education Authority, Alison Coe and Sandy, my cat.

The publishing team who came to Chartres, and were a wonderful support: Jo Godfrey Wood, Susanna Abbott, Lucy Guenot, Suzie Boston and Lynn Bresler.

My dance teachers and guides: Maria-Gabriele Wosien, June Watts, Wolfgang Larcher, Ruth White.

Publisher's acknowledgments

Gaia Books would like to thank Jeff Saward for extensive help with the Resources and consultation; Robert Ferré for writing the foreword and consultation; Peter Dawkins, the Zoence Academy and Siegfried Prumbach for information on lines of earth energy; Ann Lewin for her poem "Jeu d'Esprit" on pp. 50–51 from *Candles and Kingfishers*; Marla Visser for her poem "A New Day" on p. 74 from *Images: women in transition*, Highland, USA; Helena Petre; and the British Library.

Thanks also to Naomi, Eleanor, Rosie and Megan Teague, Sylvain, Emma and Paul Guenot, Helena Petre, Sue Haynes, Helen Conway Jones, and Sylvia Pearson for modelling and providing invaluable help with the photography. Thanks to Owen and Jenny Dixon for design help.

Photographic and illustration credits

pp.2, 8, 10, 12–13 (background photo), 14–15 (background photo), 40, 44–45, 47, 60, 63 (top), 65 (bottom), 66, 68–69, 72–73, 74–75, 76–77, 79, 80–81, 84–85, 86–87, 90–91, 94–95, 98–99, 106, Steve Teague; pp.5, 7, 11, 18–19, 23, 27, 28 (photos and drawing), 30 (top), 31, 32 (top right), 34–35, 37, 38, 42 (top left), 43 (bottom right), 53, 57, 67, 92–93, 104, Jeff Saward; p.9, David Noton; p.52, Michael Malyszko; p.62 (left and right), Thomas Wiewandt, Telegraph Colour Library; pp.14, 30 (bottom), 32 (bottom and left), Janet and Colin Bord/Fortean Picture Library; pp.15 (bottom), 17, 46, Mark Preston; pp.16, 61 (top), Robert Gutsell; pp.20, 62 (middle), Sonia Halliday and Laura Lushington; p.21, BBC Natural History Unit, © Naturbild; pp.24, 25 (top right and left, and bottom right), Science Photo Library; p.25 (bottom left), David Cavagnaro; p.29 (bottom right), Bibliothèque Nationale de Paris, Collection Scheffer; p.33 (right), Super Stock; p.36, Hereford Cathedral Library, © The Dean and Chapter of Hereford Cathedral and the Hereford Mappa Mundi Trust; p.41, K. Collins, p.55 (top), Mark Hamblin, p.55 (left), Steve Austin, Woodfall Wild Images; p.55 (bottom), Alan Watson/Forest light; pp.13 (top), 42–43 (middle three shots), 48 (top), 50–51, 63 (bottom), supplied by the author with thanks to June Hyde and Austin Winkley; pp.58–59, 61 (bottom), 65 (left), Nick Halpin, University of Dundee; p.65 (right), Ronald Sheridan, Ancient Art and Architecture; pp.70–71 Museo Nazionale, Naples.

For further information on labyrinths and forthcoming workshops you can contact the author at:
helenraphael@hotmail.com